Cancer: Exploring YOUR Path

Teresa K. Matthews

Teresa Matthews

Cancer: Exploring YOUR Path

© 2017 Teresa Matthews

Print ISBN: 978-1-54390-775-9

eBook ISBN: 978-1-54390-776-6

Dedicated to Joan Kalvelage Miller
and Siusiadh Rasmussen,
who showed me the way,
and to my beloved husband Joe,
who is with me every step of the journey

TABLE OF CONTENTS

Attitude

The longer I live, the more I realize the impact of attitude on life. Attitude, to me, is more important than facts. It is more important than education, than money, than circumstances, than failures, than successes, than what other people think or say or do. It is more important than appearance, giftedness, or skill. It will make or break a company . . . a church . . . a home. The remarkable thing is we have a choice every day regarding the attitude we will embrace for that day. We cannot change the past. We cannot change the fact that people will act a certain way. We cannot change the inevitable. The only thing we can do is play on the one string we have, and that is our attitude. I am convinced that life is 10% what happens to me and 90% how I react to it. And so it is with you . . . we are in charge of our attitudes.

—Charles Swindall in *Grace Notes,* Monroe Louisiana
From *The Anglican Digest, Advent A. D. 1992*

PART I

Cancer: The Adventure of Your Life!

Introduction

Why in the world would I write *another* self-help book about cancer? So many people's lives, not just mine, have been touched with this challenge. So many other books are on the market, profound books, scholarly books, spiritual books, scientific books. What is different here?

For one thing, I felt a burning need to write about my experiences and acquired wisdom as a part of my own healing and growth. I recovered, and I want to share what worked for me! For another, the advice I have received and in turn passed on has made a dramatic difference in my life and the lives of fellow cancer patients. Sometimes the most helpful tip seems almost humble in terms of "significance"— numbing the area with ice or a spray before a needle stick. These are the things I wish I had known when I needed them and found out along the way. My degree in biology, my work as a hospice volunteer, and a high level of familiarity with medicine should have prepared me to deal with my own illness, but I was devastated! If I felt so overwhelmed, how would someone unfamiliar with medical routines and jargon feel? In sharing my experiences with you, I hope to ease your path.

In the fall of 1994 I was a normal, active, fortyish mom with three teenage children and a husband who worked long, demanding hours. I was organized, intense, and driven by to-do lists. My life was full—*very* full. Twinges of abdominal pain led me to the doctor, and in November 1994 I was diagnosed with ovarian cancer. I spent about a week getting various diagnostic tests before major surgery in my own town. Several weeks after the surgery, I began chemotherapy. A "second look" surgery (the standard of care at the time) was performed at a regional cancer center after completion of treatment. The surgery showed no sign of cancer, and I completed chemotherapy treatments by the end of 1995. In January 1997, an abnormal mammogram and a biopsy revealed breast cancer, unrelated to my ovarian cancer. A mastectomy was performed in February, followed by chemotherapy and radiation treatments.

I am delighted to be free of clinical evidence of cancer as I write—July, 2017. Being a twenty-three-year survivor of ovarian cancer and a twenty-year survivor of breast cancer is a continuing thrill. I am watched carefully by my gynecologist but I currently live a very happy life and am able to do just about anything I want to do.

Nothing gave me more hope during my cancer time than meeting survivors, both men and women. In the last twenty-three years I have been privileged to talk with hundreds of other cancer patients. Many have urged me to write down the small tips and large outlooks that have helped us. I want to help you be a survivor who can embrace life.

Certainly with cancer, as with life, "to everything there is a season." The newly diagnosed woman with breast cancer who is deciding between a lumpectomy and a mastectomy is not helped by the story of the man who just had a bone marrow transplant. Although knowledge is power, too much knowledge—or the wrong kind of information when your resources are already overwhelmed—is discouraging rather than uplifting. What does help is to know you are not alone and not crazy! You need access to specific answers to the questions that are foremost on your mind right now and practical self-care tips for each stage of the journey.

I hope you will use this book in an unusual way. Rather than reading the book straight through like a story or a how-to book, use the book as a reference for those times when you have a specific area of concern. Our lives are challenged enough by the treatments that are directly before us. You don't need to take on the worries of tomorrow that may never even need to be faced. I urge you to use this book the way you would use a conversation with a trusted friend. Seek counsel for the immediate problem and leave the long-term concerns for a time when they require attention. Take comfort from the knowledge that you will not be left without resources when you need them in the future. If you just want a quick overview of a chapter, refer to the summary points at the end of that discussion.

Because cancer is actually a unique disease in each person, and because each body and each treatment plan are different in their details, Part I of this book is divided into general concerns for cancer patients and specific treatment modalities. Part II addresses the concerns of patients who face living with cancer long term. The ultimate judge of each suggestion in the book is your own intelligence and the advice of your healing team. No comment is intended to undermine the central role your physicians must play in your health care. I have made every effort to be sure the medical comments in the book are factual. Thankfully research continues and new discoveries may make our present coping techniques obsolete.

Sit back. Relax. Grab a cup of tea or a glass of lemonade, and come and journey with me.

The Big C

In our modern world nothing so inspires fear as the word "cancer." A recent survey showed that a cancer diagnosis is more feared than natural calamities such as earthquakes, accidents in a car or airplane, loss of a job, or loss of a spouse. With this in mind, and given that about one in three of us will be diagnosed with cancer sometime in our lifetime, it is not surprising that our hearts plummet to our shoes when we hear that we have cancer. Our culture sees youth, long life, good looks, and good health as universal goals. Obviously cancer, which disrupts all these goals, must be a monster to be feared.

When you hear the words "The pathology report shows that you have cancer," your immediate reaction is to stop listening and to go into shock. It really doesn't matter what else the doctor has to say. You are not interested in statistics, treatment plans, level of severity of the disease, or even the next step to take. Your life, as you knew it, *is* over, because from now on everything you do will be tempered with this knowledge. That is not to say that this new life will be worse. In fact, I firmly believe that this diagnosis may be one of the most powerful forces for good in your entire life. Suddenly you are at a crossroads. You can continue as if nothing has changed and push away the boogeymen that crowd your consciousness, clamoring with one shout louder than the next: "Hair loss!" "Costs!" "Children!" "Job!" "Pain!" and the most frightening one of all, "I am going to die!" Or you can begin to grapple with this opportunity for a quantum leap of perspective to a new view of life.

In point of fact, you *are* going to die. So is everyone else in this world. The difference is that now you see death as a personal threat rather than a vague, mysterious concept that applies to others but not you. When you hear the word "cancer," it galvanizes you to respond. This book will suggest a variety of positive, helpful responses that can overcome fear and self-pity and lead you to joy.

Cancer comes in a staggering variety of kinds, stages, levels of severity, and prognoses. It is difficult to write a generic "coping with cancer" book. If you have been diagnosed with a skin cancer that was completely removed at the first biopsy with little chance of recurrence, you will be in a very different place from the person who is terminally ill with metastatic cancer. What does generalize, however, is the kind of treatment that is often used for cancers today, the side effects, and the coping strategies.

In Part I you will find general wellness suggestions for anyone, with a special emphasis on known ways to strengthen our immune system (the body's own internal defense against cancer) and those that increase our sense of participation in our own good health. Following are chapters about specific treatments and their side effects, focusing on advice you need "in the trenches."

Cancer patients often learn, to their surprise, that their biggest challenge is not physical but psychological. Pain can be medicated, surgery can be performed, chemotherapy can be given. The truth is that only the patient himself or herself can seek to resolve the issues of control (and lack thereof!) that are such a stressful part of the disease process. Many of us are classic "type A" people, busy giving directions, making plans, caring for others, and sacrificing our own needs in the process. It is profoundly humbling to realize with stark clarity that we are in control of nothing. We cannot count on force of will and years of experience to keep us safe from our own mortality.

And if we are not in control of our life (as we are not), we are most certainly not in control of the details of our lives. Part of the shock of the initial diagnosis is the realization that date books painstakingly filled with plans for the next three months of our lives will be irrelevant, maybe permanently. No longer can we say, "I'll have that project done by next Friday." Suddenly our lives are scheduled around an opening in the surgeon's schedule, a daily radiation appointment, or a chemotherapy date. We don't stop living our old lives, but we must now consider each action we take, each promise we make, in light of the reality that our cancer has an effect. Like the old rose-colored glasses, cancer-colored glasses shape the way we see everything. What initially seems a distortion, will, in time, become our new reality. We can choose to become stronger and healthier by far than we were.

But you are the director of this play—you are the leader of your own journey, and you have the final decision to make. You can "get back to normal" and return to your old routines and point of view, or you can divide your life into time B.C. (before cancer) and A.D. (after diagnosis). I am convinced that the lessons of this journey are far too important to be left behind when they are no longer needed for daily survival. The gift of this new life perspective is joy.

You have the power to choose. Are you going to be known as a person dying of *cancer*? Or as a person *living* (who just happens to have cancer)? The choice you make will touch every aspect of your future, so consider it well.

In short:

- Cancer is not one disease, but many.

- It is a life-changing experience.

- Read Chapters 1-11 for general information (see the tips at the end of each chapter).

- Read Chapters 12-21 for treatment-specific helps.

- Read Part II if you are dealing with cancer as a chronic condition.

What is Cancer, Anyway?

✿❦✿

Because the word is tossed around so frequently you may be shy about asking, "What *is* this disease?" It may seem everyone knows but you. Don't be alarmed. It is possible to understand some basic facts without jumping into a sea of medical terminology that can be intimidating, to say the least.

In the beginning, every human being starts as two cells which combine—the egg from the mother and the sperm from the father. The resulting embryo grows, and as it does, the number of cells increases. Each embryonic cell splits into two offspring cells, over and over again. Not only does the number of cells increase, but the cells begin to take on particular characteristics, depending on their future site and use in the body. At birth, a baby has dozens of different cell types, each tailor-made for a specific function. These cells are organized into tissues (collections of cells with similar functions) and organs. Each organ or gland (breast, pancreas, liver, prostate, or colon) contains several cell types. It is an amazing system that works—without any action from us— to allow us to eat, run, breathe, think, circulate our blood, and reproduce. All in all, quite a huge task!

In the course of normal life, as cells grow old or are lost through friction, illness, or injury, the body replaces those cells by producing new offspring cells of the same type. An intricate system is in place at the cellular level to provide "brakes" for cell division, so that only as many new cells as are needed are produced. In the case of cancer, this normal braking function is not in place, so cell reproduction continues out of control.

What causes a normal cell to lose its inhibitions and become cancerous? Researchers all over the world are looking for that answer. We know some causes of cancer, but in most cases a combination of several risk factors is at work. For example, we know that smoking or smokeless tobacco causes cell damage that can lead to cancer. Some people are born with cells that already are genetically susceptible to cancer, which is why your doctor will ask you if any relatives have cancer. The chemicals called carcinogens have been tested and shown to produce cancer in animals or people. Radiation can lead to an increased risk of cancer, as evidenced in the survivors of the nuclear attacks in Japan. Sun damage can lead to skin cancer.

The body normally responds to "mutant" or damaged cells by destroying them. Specialized cells in the bloodstream, part of our immune system, recognize the cancer cells as foreign and attack and kill them. Unfortunately the number of cancer cells can overwhelm the system, or the cancer cells may be disguised to avoid this first line of defense.

Whatever the combination of causes, a single cell begins to divide without the usual controls. As more and more offspring cells are produced, a tumor is formed. A tumor is a collection of cancerous cells. The kind of tumor that results will depend on the initial faulty cell. For example, a basal-cell carcinoma begins with a basal cell in the skin, and a ductal carcinoma of the breast grows from a cell normally found in the ducts of the breast. In the beginning, the group of cells forming the tumor remains near the original cell. If the tumor is not removed or treated, it will continue to grow. Some tumors are benign, which means that they will never travel to distant parts of the body. They grow by pushing normal tissue away. Benign tumors can still be a problem, however, if their growth pushes on other organs.

A malignant tumor (cancer), on the other hand, grows as cancer cells actually mingle with the normal cells that surround them. It begins as a small group of cells in just one region. Doctors call this "carcinoma *in situ*," which means that the tumor is still in a relatively small area. When the cancer begins to show up in surrounding cells it is called "invasive."

As cancerous cells continue to divide, some cells may break away from the original tumor site and travel through the body, sometimes to settle in distant areas and start new tumors there. If that happens, the patient is said to have "metastatic" cancer. The cancerous cells that move away from the site will carry with them the characteristics of the original faulty cell. A ductal breast cancer will continue to look, microscopically, like breast cancer even if it has traveled to the lymph nodes, brain, or liver. In fact, it *is* still breast cancer and is likely to be treated by chemotherapy and radiation the way the original tumor is treated. Leukemia, sometimes called cancer of the blood, is actually uncontrolled growth of certain blood cells produced in the bone marrow.

A pathologist will examine your own particular cancer to determine not only what kind of cell is involved but also how fast the cells are dividing, how far they have invaded into surrounding normal tissues, and whether or not the tumor has spread to distant parts of the body. Your tumor will be described in technical terms on your pathology report, and this accurate description is the basis for your personalized treatment regimen.

Surgery, radiation, and much chemotherapy are aimed at either killing or removing the cancerous cells. Treatments to prevent the cancer cells from multiplying can provide protection on a long-term basis. The breast cancer drugs Tamoxifen and Arimidex are examples of drugs used for this purpose.

Both radiation and chemotherapy tend to be non-specific. They work by killing cells that are in the process of dividing. In most cases the dividing cells are the cancerous ones. Some of the normal cells in the body are also constantly dividing as part of their function, for instance the cells lining the mouth and stomach, the cells of the skin, and the blood cells. The oncologist (a doctor who specializes in treating cancer) tries to design a therapy that will have the maximum effect on the cancer with the least impact on the normal cells that surround it.

Researchers hope to discover much more specific tools in the future. One promising area of research involves drugs "tailor-made" for each tumor to seek out only those cells. Other investigators hope to be able to use genetic testing to predict which people are at high risk of developing a particular cancer. Some potential treatments would improve the efficiency of our "early warning system" to detect and destroy tumor cells. Research continues into drugs that can interfere with the formation of blood vessels in tumors. Certainly this is a hopeful time to be living with cancer. We are seeing an explosion of new information and specific treatments.

In short:

- Cancer refers to a group of diseases characterized by uncontrolled cell growth.

- The site of the first cancerous cell determines what that cancer is called, even if the same cancer shows up in a distant part of the body.

- Most cancer treatments are aimed at rapidly dividing cells and may kill some normal "innocent bystander" cells, too.

Psychological Impacts

The impact of a cancer diagnosis certainly varies from person to person, but it always includes a sense of vulnerability and lack of control. For people with life-threatening cancer, there is also a very real sense of loss, the loss of one's own good health and perhaps the loss of a body part, of a job, or of the ability to perform the usual routines. As with any loss, grief is a part of the process of recovery and getting on with one's new life.

Initially it takes about three weeks for the reality of illness to sink in to our consciousness. The mind shifts gears, as it were, to see the self in a new way. This first three weeks can seem like time in a dream, with a sense of unreality and an inability to focus thoughts clearly. Even during that time, however, the elements of grief can be present in varying degrees. I found myself bursting into tears for no reason at all and unable to concentrate or process information (especially about my cancer).

Grief is a process that each person handles in his or her own unique way, but it usually includes the following stages. Denial says, "This can't be happening to me, there has been some mistake, everything is really fine." Anger rages, "This is *so* unfair! I have always taken such good care of myself.

The doctors should have caught this sooner." Bargaining tries to reach a compromise: "If only the CT scan shows that the lung cancer is treatable, I'll never smoke another cigarette." Depression whispers, "I simply cannot face the future; if I am to be ill, what's the use?" Allowing each of these stages to be recognized and addressed can lead to final acceptance. Acceptance reasons, "If this is where I am, I guess my choice is to make the best of it." The length of time in each stage can vary from minutes to years, and the severity of the response depends on each person's experience and emotional make-up. It is important to realize that grief is part of your total wellness picture because some of the "symptoms" of grief can mask, mimic, or overshadow the physical symptoms of the cancer.

Physical symptoms of grief can include any of the following: Lack of ability to concentrate, sleep disruptions (more or less than usual), appetite disruptions (nothing tastes good or eating all the time), tearfulness, nausea, dry mouth, tremors, loss of memory, headaches, or any combination of these. It is reassuring to know that you are not losing your mind! These are normal physical responses to the overwhelming assault on your sense of self. During this time you will most likely be under close medical care, sometimes involving several medical procedures or appointments each week. It is always a good idea to let your physician know how you are feeling if you experience any of these symptoms. He or she can determine if the symptom is a result of the cancer, the treatment, or your grief process and can recommend appropriate action to make you more comfortable.

Many cancer patients find the psychological demands of dealing with cancer are more energy-requiring and more upsetting than the physical components of treatment, such as hair loss, nausea, or fatigue. A friend once commented on her mother's experience with breast cancer, "I am finally realizing that this is a battle in the mind more than in the body." Especially in a society that values health and strength and beauty as much as ours does, the loss of any of these attributes can feel like a loss of everything that is important.

Perhaps the most universal emotional response to cancer is fear. Even those folks who are bold in the face of most of life's challenges may be overcome with a fear so powerful that they feel paralyzed. The components of this fear are so many that it is difficult to cope with any one because others crowd in. You may experience fear of death, fear of hospitals, fear of pain, fear of loss of a body part, fear of loss of relationships that are valuable to you, fear of loss of courage, fear of side effects, fear of economic ruin, fear of loss of a job—the list goes on and on. We are all accustomed to dealing with fear in the normal course of our life, but usually the fear is about more trivial matters; for example, we may fear being out of place. Nothing prepares us for such a cluster of fears about so many very important issues at one time. Coping mechanisms are stretched, not only for the patient but also for the family.

Fear is always future-oriented. It's always about something that is *going to* happen or more accurately, *might* happen. It's always about the bad possibilities and leaves out the unanticipated happy surprises that you don't know about yet: friends you haven't met, books you haven't read, money you didn't expect to receive, laws that change in your favor, or the inner strength you develop. Fear is always based on life not going the way you have decided is the best/right way. If you are dealing with strong emotions about a current problem, you aren't dealing with fear, but rather are searching for coping mechanisms.

Why can't we just ignore the fear, pretend it isn't there? Most importantly, that doesn't work! Fear won't be ignored, and trying to ignore it only makes it grow. Fear uses up our mental and emotional resources and our time, and robs us of the space we want and need for hope, joy, and strength. It isn't just a neutral void within us, it is a negative filler, taking up space that is needed for what is true, good, and worthy of praise. Casting out fear is like spring cleaning.

Fears have a way of coming out of hiding at night or any time our busy "in-charge" selves let down our defenses. Somehow the fear that was awful during the day is magnified many times into intolerable and certain doom at night. Being human and wanting to avoid pain, we have a natural tendency to push the fear away. We try to sweep it under the carpet and stay too busy to let fear in at all. Actually the most helpful response is just the opposite. The most useful tool against fear is to look it right in the face and know that even if your fear comes true, you can find the courage and resources to handle it.

One effective technique, based on Cognitive Behavioral Therapy, is to choose a time during the day to do some "fear work." When you are reasonably well-rested and temporarily free of interruption or distraction, make yourself comfortable. I chose times when I was alone in the house. I would brew a cup of tea and sit with a box of tissues and a pad of yellow lined paper. Allow your mind to open the closet that holds all of your fears. One at a time, take each fear out, write it down, and name it. Is it fear of losing your job? Fear of the emotional impact on your family? Write them all down. Ask yourself if that fear came true, what would you do? What would your alternatives be? Recognize that you have options in any situation, even if the choices are acceptance in peace rather than flailing in fear. When you have worked on this list, either in one sitting or several, you can recognize at any given moment exactly which fear is immobilizing you.

When fear comes calling in the middle of the night, you can say, "I know this fear, it is the fear of pain. I have looked at it before, and I do not need to be controlled by it. Even if this comes to pass, I will still be OK. My self will not perish. Go away, fear of pain!" Does it sound corny? Sure, but it works! Certainly this is not a guarantee that you will have immediate freedom from fear, but as the process is repeated you can gain some level of comfort. Each time the fear is named it loses some of its power over you until you begin to deal with your fears with your rational mind rather than with your frightened emotions.

Another approach to the fear of cancer is a treatment called EMDR (Eye Movement Desensitation and Reprogramming). This is administered by a trained therapist who uses eye movements similar to those occurring naturally during dreaming. This treatment can help you see disturbing material in a new, less disturbing way. (For more information see EMDRIA.com.)

Control issues become evident when you become a patient. In the physical realm alone you may have no control over the scheduling of procedures, the choice of nursing personnel, or the time of your hospital meal. ("What? Breakfast at seven A.M.? But I just got to sleep, finally!") For people used to planning each day down to ten-minute intervals, this is disconcerting to say the least. On a spiritual and emotional basis, the loss of control is even more evident and upsetting. The idea that "I will take care of all those loose ends, get my life together, make a will, reconcile with my brother . . . before I die," is gone. Instead we may think, "O my gosh! What if I die tomorrow?" Suddenly we are aware that, in the final analysis, our continued existence is not up to us. We cannot *will* ourselves to escape death. We are not our own creators or healers. For me and for many others this awareness triggers intense soul-searching and moves spiritual and after-death questions from a mental "back burner" to front and center! (See Chapter 7, The Soul Perspective.)

This is not to say that we can do nothing because we can and should take an active part in our own healing. It is true, however, that even the person with the most terrific attitude may die quickly of a rapidly progressing disease, while a nasty, bitter, complaining person may linger for years and make life miserable for all around them. The final result simply isn't up to us.

Once that awareness hits, and it usually quickly follows the initial diagnosis, our challenge is deciding what to do with this loss of control. It may help to see that the reality (of not being in control) hasn't changed, only the fact that now we *understand* the reality as it applies directly to us. As I was waiting for a CT scan during the week between my initial diagnosis and the surgery, my oncologist walked by and saw me waiting, obviously distraught. I'll never forget his words to me: "This is the hardest part." I'm sure my disbelief was written all over my face. "Really," he said, "once you take the first step in the treatment plan, once you and your doctors know what it is that you are facing, a huge weight of doubt is taken off your shoulders. You can learn what factors are to be considered and participate in the decisions to be made. Each step in treatment becomes a conscious choice, to be accepted and embraced as the right thing to do. The stress comes from not knowing." My own experience and that of my friends has proved his words true. The time between the awareness of lack of control and the formation of a plan to deal with factors we *can* control is the most difficult time of all.

One part of the cancer journey that can make progress more difficult is the problem of depression. You may experience normal and temporary sadness, blues, or discouragement that are just part of the grieving process, or you may suffer from true clinical depression. If your symptoms are severe or persistent you may need professional help in the form of psychotherapy, counseling, or medication. Check with your physician. This is not a sign of weakness but an acknowledgement that your progress toward health can be aided by the tools of a professional.

On the other hand, if you have one or several "down" days, some actions you can take on your own may help. First, recognize that this is a part of the disease process. Challenges that you could take in stride before your illness may be too much to deal with if you are in a physically or emotionally depleted state. Depression is *not* a sign of weakness on your part but a real physical reaction to everything you must face. It is both OK and normal to feel sad, but it isn't the sort of attitude that is particularly pleasant or helpful. Action to lift your spirits is certainly worth a try.

What kinds of things lift spirits? As many as there are different spirits to lift! Some tried and true ways may help.

- Refer to yourself whenever possible as a person who *had* cancer, not as a person who *has* cancer. Don't let your illness redefine you as a "cancer patient." I chose to consider my cancer gone after my initial surgery and to regard all the other treatments as "insurance." I am not an ovarian cancer patient but rather a person with a history of cancer who is now busy living. This attitude—I am OK, right now—allows you to embrace life without the tentativeness of seeing yourself as an invalid.

- Make a list of everything you have to be thankful for—enough food, shelter, clothing, friends, spouse, children, sunshine, freedom, trees, whatever! Keep going as more and more ideas come to mind. This tends to lend perspective to your problems.

- Make it a point to go through the day looking for the best it has to offer. Write it down that night. It may be a leaf edged with frost or a sunset or a note from a friend or a nap. The result of this looking for good is that you find it much more often than you would expect when you are feeling low.

- Do something for someone else. Say a prayer, write a note, make a phone call, smile at a clerk. It is hard to be sad when someone else is gladdened by your presence. One chemo buddy came in several times a *week* for treatments of his leukemia. His incredible sense of joy, humor, and giving brightened the day for everyone in the room.

-Try something new. Read a new book, watch a movie, learn a new language, start a needlepoint, explore an interest. Maybe now is the time to try your hand at writing, painting, or gardening. The point is not the final product but the pleasure of the activity. You have no one to please but yourself!

- Reach out to friends for company and support. Stay connected to the relationships that are important to you. Often friends tend to stay away, not wanting to bother you or interrupt a nap. They may be eager to get together for a short visit if you make the first move. When you visit, be sure to be a good listener and express interest in what is happening in your friend's life. It is not helpful just to complain. Visitors may tend to avoid you in the future, out of a sense that they were helpless to "fix" your problems.

- If you need to vent you may want to consider a professional listener such as a priest or minister, a counselor, or a social worker. You need your friends to be *friends*. Many of my deepest fears, such as the worry that I would be too chicken to go through treatments, I did not share even with my husband because I thought that my fear would add to his burden. Venting to a professional allows you to express all of your feelings freely and clearly, without weighing words or worrying about what someone else thinks of you or whether your words will cause pain for the listener. Some factors other than depression that may indicate the need for professional help include a history of trauma, a limited or non-existent support system, despair, or collapse of primary relationships.

- Try doing again what has brought you pleasure in the past. Maybe you love the mountains—how about an afternoon drive? Perhaps you long for a gourmet meal at a fine restaurant, just like in the old days. Do it! Past sources of support can help you again.

- Talk with others who are struggling with problems in their own lives. When you ask yourself if you would rather have cancer than Alzheimer's disease, mental retardation, multiple sclerosis, deafness, or blindness, you may discover that you prefer the illness that is *your* challenge. A family friend always used to encourage us by saying, "The devil you know is better than the devil you don't know." Recognize that even the most apparently perfect life has its difficulties, although they may not be evident to you.

- Remember that the course of life in general, and cancer in particular, is a roller-coaster ride. When you are down, you can be assured that another up is around the corner, although it is difficult to see that when you are weighted down with depression. Let your past experiences of joyful times give you hope now.

In short:

- Your cancer diagnosis will have both an immediate and a delayed effect on your mind and emotions.

- Going through physical changes due to grieving is normal.

- The emotional challenge of cancer can be more depleting than the physical treatments.

- Facing your fears can bring you a measure of inner peace.

- This is an amazing experience for control freaks and an opportunity for learning how to let go.

- Depression can be helped by:

  - Counting your blessings

  - Helping someone else

  - Meeting your physical needs for regular sleep, exercise and food

  - Staying connected with friends

  - Trying something new, a hobby or interest

  - Returning to past activities that cheered you

  - Sharing experiences with others who are coping with their own problems

  - Venting to a professional counselor or other support person

  - Realizing that moods come in cycles, and a better one is just around the corner.

Cancer as a Family Affair

"What about the children?" is probably one of the most frequent responses to a cancer diagnosis. If the patient is a parent, especially if the children are still in the household, a cancer diagnosis is not just a personal challenge but definitely a family matter. On one hand, concern for children is a powerful motivator, leading many patients to say, "I'll do whatever is necessary to give me the best shot at a cure because my children need me." On the other hand, worry about the rest of the family can add additional stress to a patient with coping resources already spread thin. The fact remains: Like it or not, cancer is a family issue.

My oncologist gave me some good advice as we discussed treatment plans at our first meeting. Without any comment from me, he said, "Don't you stop being a mother! Your daughter needs you to be her mom, now more than ever." (My daughter was thirteen, and my two sons were away at college.) I was surprised by his remark until I realized what I had been thinking. "If I only have a short while to spend with my daughter, I want that to be top-quality time. Maybe I shouldn't insist on homework getting done. I really don't want to waste time by making her do chores. We could take trips together . . ." In fact, as my doctor pointed out, the best way to help children cope with the cancer of their parent is to continue being the parent! Cancer therapy consumes a lot of time and energy, and the routines and schedules of a busy family are usually disrupted in a major way. In the midst of having our "usual" ways thrown out the window, the last thing a child needs is a parent who changes all the family rules and roles. I was lucky to get this warning at the start. It saved me from making mistakes I would have regretted.

In fact, our task as parents is no different when cancer is a part of the family from what it was before the illness. Our goal is to raise self-assured, confident, and competent individuals equipped to function independently in a complex world. Cancer simply moves the timetable up, so our children learn earlier than their peers to ask what really matters in life. It is a normal parenting desire to protect those we love from pain. In the real world, however, it is impossible to avoid pain, and coming to grips with difficulty early in life can often result in children who are much more mature than their peers and much more flexible in dealing with unexpected disappointments or changes of plans.

What tools can we use to help our families through the challenge that is cancer? The most important, most necessary key to maintaining healthy family relationships is honesty. Although it seems overwhelming to an adult, cancer of a parent can feel even more devastating to a child, as though her own life is over. Children, too, experience loss—the loss of the illusion that parents have all the answers, will always be available, and are immortal. The reality, no matter how difficult, is always better than the scenarios that are created in the active imagination of a child. The way to help your children the most is to give them, without exception, the information that they ask for.

After our initial meeting with the oncologist, when we did have a "battle plan" in place, we had a family meeting. We told them everything we knew about the kind of cancer involved, the location, the type of surgery and the surgery results, and the plan for chemotherapy. Then we answered questions. The rule was, "No question is too trivial or too personal. If you are wondering, *ask* us." We sat and talked for several hours, going into all of the nuts and bolts of family life. Who will drive the carpool? Will we be able to afford my tuition? Who will do the dishes and cook? Can you still come to my concerts? Will you die? Some of the questions were straightforward and others required us to find out the answers. Some simply were unanswerable. We all left that day, however, knowing that we were in this together and promising that we would not keep secrets from one another. As treatments unfolded, we made it a point to let each person know what was happening.

As it turned out, each of my sons decided to take some time out from his demanding college course of study to return home for a few months. They found that they could not concentrate on school while wondering about how I was doing. It was much more important to them to be with me. Their time at home was precious family time, a gift from them and also a gift to them. Somehow staying on an arbitrary class schedule was not as critical as doing what their heart urged them to do. (Amazingly both finished college in four years in spite of realigning their priorities!)

Just as flexibility is required from the patient, who may not be able to predict a good day or a bad day, the family learns to be flexible. For example, what if your chemo treatment is scheduled for the day before Thanksgiving? Maybe this year the family can go to an uncle's home for dinner. Maybe you'll celebrate a week early. Maybe you'll change the treatment date. The key is that everyone's needs are considered and that the family recognizes everyone is working together to meet those needs. At the same time, family traditions are important. If possible, try to continue with activities such as cutting down your Christmas tree or going camping together, whatever is meaningful for *your* family.

What about your spouse? This life-mate, this person who promised to live with you "for better or worse, in sickness and in health, as long as you both shall live" is now faced with a future that includes uncertainty, sickness, and maybe disability or death. It is inconceivable. The spouse of someone with cancer is faced with a perplexing array of problems. The logistics of dividing family chores and caregiving roles is staggering. Their beloved friend who has always been available to offer support after a hard day may now be the one who *needs* support at the end of the day. The patient may not have the energy to continue in-home or outside jobs. Financial concerns can be huge. The spouse is suddenly faced with a greatly increased workload at the same time his or her own emotional reserves are being depleted by worry. There is no single solution, but three common threads of resolve seem to characterize the marriages that survive and thrive.

You, the patient, must take charge of your own health. That commitment can ease the burden greatly for your spouse. Often the things necessary for recovery are not much fun: drinking lots of fluids, getting out for exercise, or eating when you'd rather not. It helped me to realize the frustration my husband felt when he knew I needed to eat but chose not to. I discovered that taking care of myself was my most important contribution to our marriage. My husband, on the other hand, realized that although he could *want* me to choose the healthiest course and *encourage* me to do so, ultimately only I could decide to take care of me. In many ways the role of the spouse is more difficult than that of the cancer patient, who is actively *doing*. The spouse must be content to provide support without patronizing or treating the patient like a child. It is a difficult job.

Secondly, the spouse can help preserve his or her own sanity in several ways. The biggest difference can result from the conscious decision to simplify life in whatever large or small ways are possible. My dear husband decided to cut back on his work schedule to allow time to be with me, to help with the hard times and celebrate the good ones. This is the time to step back from extra commitments, from outside activities, from striving for perfection. Any time and energy that can be saved will replenish the reserves that are used for care giving. This is also an important time to connect with old or new friends who will allow venting or emotional support. The spouse needs to be able to talk freely with someone who is removed from the immediate family and can listen without being hurt, making judgments, or giving advice. It is particularly helpful to talk with someone who has been in a similar position, to be reassured that feelings of frustration and irritation are normal and do not signify a lack of love. Even (especially!) in the midst of treatments, it is important for the spouse to make time to get away, to seek respite and refreshment by being alone.

The third coping mechanism for the spouse of a cancer patient is to become involved in the journey. Learning about the disease facing you helps both partners to understand the particular aspects of treatment that are most difficult for the patient. The more your spouse knows, the easier it will be for him or her to be supportive and non-judgmental. For example, maybe the husband is a shy person who will not ask questions or ask for help, even when faced with the unknown of chemotherapy treatment. It may help a lot for his wife to come along for chemo treatments to relay questions, ask for a warm blanket, or just be a comforting presence. Perhaps the wife is struggling with aching muscles following a treatment. If her husband knows that, he can be especially gentle with a hug. The spouse can find out what days are hardest for the patient and surprise him or her with a new CD of a favorite music group, a single flower, or a comfort meal.

Expect challenges to your sexual relationship. Cancer treatments may deplete energy, can cause physical distress, and will change body image. Some medications can impact sexual desire. A healthy sexuality can do a lot to support your immune system, improve emotional closeness, and restore hope and joy. It is worth the trouble to explore options if you are struggling in this area.

Many aspects of the family culture change during treatment for cancer. If Mom has always done the shopping, cooking, and dishes, this may be a good time to change habits. Perhaps the kids just casually leave their shoes, clothes, toys, or books wherever they fall. Does the phone ring all evening with conversations between buddies? I found that my tolerance for confusion, disorder, and cleaning up after others plummeted. I was easily overwhelmed. I was frustrated that I needed to deal with unnecessary stresses when the challenge of getting well took all of my energy and attention. My solution was to draw up a set of boundaries for my family and me. My list included these.

- Each person is responsible for removing his belongings from the common family living space.

- I will be unavailable for any non-emergency needs after eight P.M. (I wasn't necessarily in bed, but I was resting and unavailable for stressful decision-making, heavy-duty thinking, or anything that would interfere with my ability to be calm enough to go to sleep.)

- No incoming phone calls after nine P.M.

- Some days, I just need silence. I can't handle loud music or TV then.

- On particularly hard days (chemo treatment days or surgery recovery time) I may not want to be around anyone. If I go into my bedroom and close the door, please understand that I still love you. Sometimes, though, I am using all of my resources just to *be,* and I have nothing left over even for a conversation. (Few days were this difficult, but it was an emotional safety net for me to know I had this option.)

Most families will adapt to the new demands and be glad for the clarity of what to expect. They will feel less helpless and frustrated if they know how to help you. If you are unwilling to talk to your family about your needs and expectations, perhaps a friend could sit down with all of you and act as a mediator.

For many families, the time around cancer can be both the most demanding and the most life-giving time spent together. Once you get past the obvious "I can't believe this is happening to my family!" you can get on with finding the many blessings you might have missed in the rush of being a "normal" family.

What if you are facing cancer alone? Cancer does not discriminate. Some folks have the support they need ready-made, all around them, coming out of the woodwork. There are also men and women in less fortunate circumstances, working because they have no choice, raising children alone while dealing with treatments, time-stressed and financially stressed. Cancer can feel like the final straw in a life that is already struggling. If this is your circumstance, what can you do?

The first step is to recognize that your emotional stability will be greatly enhanced by gathering one or more caring people around you. This is an extremely tough road to walk alone. Just saying, "I'm doing fine, I'll be OK on my own," doesn't make it so. You can do yourself a huge favor by seeking connections with others. It is a gift to them, too, to be able to help.

Where do you find these support people? Often they are already present in your life in a peripheral way (grown siblings or cousins, for example). Check your address book. Check your Christmas card list. Consider your social media friends. Your church leaders or outreach workers can offer experienced and caring counsel and specific assistance as needed. Sometimes these folks will come to you when they hear you are ill and will take the initiative to bring meals, send cards, or phone you. More often you will need to seek their help by making your illness and your needs known. Potential helpers may keep their distance out of respect for your privacy. If you can invite them to help or give them permission to participate with you, you may discover a new, clearer focus to your relationship. Most potential support people are glad to be of assistance, just as you would be honored and willing to help someone else.

Another excellent source of support is your medical team. Your doctors, infusion nurses, or radiation techs will often know a survivor who has faced challenges similar to your own. It is unlikely that they will volunteer this information, but if you ask about finding a mentor they may be willing to check with past patients and set up a phone contact. The majority of cancer survivors remember their own struggles and are willing, even eager, to do what they can to help others.

Take advantage of the resources available to every person with cancer.

- The American Cancer Society and the National Cancer Institute both have 24-hour help lines, free (see bibliography). They also offer on-line support. Your own particular type of cancer may qualify you for specific help. There are dedicated professionals, free materials by mail for the asking, and experienced volunteers who can suggest insider tips for dealing with things like lymphoma, leukemia, prostate cancer, and breast cancer.

- Many hospitals offer support groups of one kind or another, either specific for cancer patients or for those dealing with serious illness in general. If you attend one or two meetings you may find that the group is an excellent place to make connections and share both concerns and triumphs. Even if you decide that the group setting isn't for you, perhaps you will meet one or two individuals who have the potential to be friends. You can set up a coffee date and get to know each other better. Having someone to call, just to chat, is worth the effort it takes to make a new friend.

- Consider using social media like Facebook or Craigslist. You can enter your "needs" and see what is available, and maybe make new friends in the process. Check out Timebank International membership.

- Need a phone? You may be able to get one for free by contacting local cell phone providers.

- Services may be available locally for rides to treatment (even including air trips to distant treatment centers) or for assistance with gas or lodging costs.

- Pharmaceutical companies may offer free or greatly discounted medications and chemotherapy in cases of financial need.

- Make friends with the people in the billing office where you receive treatments. They are professionals at figuring out the best way to help you with financial matters. They will often make phone calls to your insurance company or Medicaid provider to see what is possible. In case of hardship, they may adjust your bill by writing off some of the cost or arranging for payments over time.

Your best source of contact with these folks is the social worker affiliated with the place you get your treatment—services are usually at no charge. They can also recommend a counselor who is experienced with patients in your situation who offers a sliding scale of fees.

Use affirmations wherever you are to remind yourself of the thing you do have control over—your attitude. Say to yourself, "I am strong and willing to fight. I will grow through this. My example can be a force for good in the lives of those around me, including my medical caregivers." Write your own affirmation and repeat it until it is a part of you.

Give yourself credit for just "showing up" for the treatments you need, which is much more difficult when you don't have a cheerleader. Be your own best encourager. Recognize both the difficulty of the journey and your own resourcefulness. You have faced challenges before and you are still here, still engaged in the hard work of seeking your best life.

If you feel alone, ask yourself if you are giving others permission to help you. Do you always say, "I'm fine, thanks," even when you aren't? We must make the choice to put ourselves in the position of receiving. It takes both a conscious decision and effort. Can you meet the challenge to allow yourself to be taken care of? Make a little room in your heart to receive love!

Whether your family is a biological one or a "found" one, you will find yourself not wanting to "impose." In fact, people of all ages can and should learn how to care for others. One of the gifts of having cancer is that the people who know you will learn from you. They will learn what is really important in your life and theirs. They will learn that often the greatest gift is the willingness to receive help from another. Most of all, they will learn that their kind and thoughtful actions do make a difference and be motivated to continue to live as generous members of society. If you refuse to ask for help, you deprive friends and family members of the chance to learn these profound lessons.

My greatest concern was that my cancer would disrupt my children's normal lives. Yes, they did grow up quickly. Our daughter, as a high school freshman, couldn't believe her classmates were so immature that they had belching contests! She had a different focus at that time in her life. As a result of our family's cancer experience, however, today they are sensitive, caring, and compassionate individuals who understand what matters to them.

In short:

- Your illness will have an impact on those you love.
- Honesty is the key to maintaining healthy relationships with people of any age.
- Flexibility can ease many of the changes in household routine.
- You can help your family most by taking good care of your own health needs.
- Respect the needs of your caregivers for emotional support and respite time away from you.
- Set reasonable guidelines for the household to preserve

good will and minimize disruption.

- If you are living alone, gather supporting friends through recommendations from medical care providers, the American Cancer Society, support groups, or your church or neighbors. Try the excellent on-line support groups.

- Allow others to help you, as a gift to both of you.

If You Are a Friend or Loved One of a Cancer Patient

How can someone who has never had a serious disease support a cancer patient? As hard as it is to be ill and dealing with the emotional, physical, and spiritual demands of this disease, at least as the patient we are the one *doing* the dealing with. Sometimes all loved ones can do is feel helpless. What can friends and family members do to help during the cancer journey? You may want to copy this chapter for people who want to know how to help you.

First of all, realize that some things are *unhelpful*. Probably the single most unhelpful thing you can do is to share any horror stories you have heard about any other cancer patient. There is *no* value in sharing that your Aunt Minnie had radiation treatments and almost died or that your neighbor "just had tumors all over her body." It is equally unhelpful to say, "You look terrible!" even if it is true. This kind of comment tends to be thrown out by someone who is ill at ease and doesn't know what to say but is desperate to say something. Saying nothing is highly preferable to saying something harmful. I would define harmful as anything that adds to the patient's sense of anxiety or alarm. Usually the patient already struggles constantly with the anxieties he or she cannot escape. The danger in telling horror stories is that the well person often assumes a correlation between the person in the story and the listener. This is absolutely false. Each person who has cancer is an individual with a different tumor, different genetics, different current health and health history. The kinds and doses of treatment are unique to that individual patient. Please bite your tongue, leave the room, or talk about the weather, but *don't* tell horror stories.

An additional reason horror stories can be harmful is that many cancer patients are consciously choosing to focus their attention on maximizing their chances for being healed of the disease. It can be both alarming and psychologically harmful to be faced, for example, with the "statistics" about survival rates for a certain type of cancer. In general a far more helpful attitude for the patient is: "It really doesn't matter what the statistics are. I am determined to do all I can to be in the percentage of patients who do exceptionally well. If I am cancer-free, the outcome for me is 100 percent positive." Statistics can cause so much harm that they are much better left to the patient and his or her doctor, *if* the patient wants this information.

The second unhelpful thing you can do is to throw out advice. "Have you tried blue-green algae?" "My friend got lots of help from a macrobiotic diet." "You should try acupuncture." Rest assured that the cancer patient has spent an incredible amount of time considering the best treatments for him- or herself and has arrived at a place where he or she feels the best treatment is the one he or she is getting. The input from several doctors (oncologist, surgeon, radiation oncologist, pathologist) and lots of reading is overwhelming enough. It takes a lot of time and emotional energy to deal with this information overload. Don't make it any worse by throwing in your pet cure. If you have had personal experience with something that has helped you or a loved one, it is OK to mention that in one sentence or so, with the question, "Would you like to hear more?" If the patient says no, *stop*. You have opened the door. When and if the time is right, the patient can take the initiative to ask you for more information.

The third demoralizing thing you can say to a cancer patient is, "I know just how you feel. I remember when I had the flu . . ." Please realize that none of us *ever* knows just how someone else feels. It is particularly upsetting to hear this when you are barely hanging on to your sanity during an especially bad time and a well-meaning friend compares your misery with something trivial. Even if you have had chemo or radiation or surgery yourself, you *still* don't know how the patient feels because each of us has a different pain threshold and reaction to treatments. A better comment is, "I can't know how you feel, but when I was going through this, I felt . . ." Then the patient is able to either let your comment stand alone or say, "Yes, I feel that way too." The difference is that you are not placing yourself in the role of an authority about something you have no way of knowing.

Don't pry. Don't be nosy. Allow the patient to discuss as much or as little of her experience with treatments or anything else as she is comfortable sharing, and consider the remarks made to you as confidential. Make a commitment to keep these things to yourself, as a sacred trust. By acting responsibly and remaining silent, you show respect for the patient and also help to prevent rumors from starting.

Don't ever speak in the patient's presence as if he can't hear you. Even if he appears to be asleep or in a coma, you might be unpleasantly surprised at the powerful impact your careless words can have. Be respectful.

Don't avoid the person because you are ill at ease or never know what to say. Your friendship is a valuable asset at this time of great turmoil, and you are needed! At least send a card or note saying you are thinking of him.

A note about cards: Be sure that if the patient may *not* be getting well, you don't send a card that says, "Get well soon." If I am looking ahead to a year of radiation and chemo treatments, a "Hurry up and get well" card only makes me think the person sending it has no clue about my life now or my feelings. Look for cards that express care without the automatic assumption that this is an illness someone will get over quickly, as if they had a cold or an appendectomy. "Thinking of you" cards are good choices or "Missing you" if that is appropriate or something humorous, if that's your style. Read the card from the point of view of the person who will receive it, and *think*.

Don't expect to be thanked. Energy resources are spread so thin there may not be time, energy, or concentration for a call or note. Consider yourself thanked silently, and know that you made a kind difference.

Now, what *does* help someone who is dealing with cancer?

- Be available but not intrusive. It is best to let the patient decide when he or she has the emotional energy and physical reserves for a phone call or a visit. Don't just show up. Don't be offended if your phone call is at a bad time. Some kinds of attention are always welcome. On my worst days, the high point of the day was getting the mail and finding a card with a brief note of concern. I loved the people who said, "Call me when you feel up to it." I appreciated flowers, teddy bears, or good luck charms for the sentiments they represented, but almost always the most important part of the support was the written or spoken word of care and concern and not the gift. Take the time and trouble to put your thoughts and your love into writing. That card will continue to bring joy each time it is reopened, and it will be!

- If you want to visit, ask the person who is ill. Say, "I'd like to see you. Is there a time that is good for you? How long should my visit be so that I don't tire you? Please tell me when you need to rest so that I can leave." This patient is working, working on getting well. The primary task of people with cancer is to take care of themselves, not entertain others. Sometimes five or ten minutes will be all the patient can handle that day. You can help by providing a graceful way for your friend to avoid the embarrassment of having to ask you to leave.

When you do visit, let the patient direct the time spent together. Ask what he wants to do. Maybe he wants you to read to him. Maybe he wants to talk without interruption, to release frustration or to vent. Maybe she wants to go for a walk or "escape" to a movie or DVD or share a special food (her choice, not yours!). And be prepared for changes in plans. It is often difficult to predict how the patient will be feeling from hour to hour or day to day, so be flexible if a nap is suddenly a higher priority than your planned visit. Be grateful that your relationship is strong enough that the patient feels free to be honest with you about his or her needs and trusts you to understand.

Realize that things may not be the same between you. The patient is dealing with tremendous changes within his own life, and that impacts how he relates to everyone else. You may need to back off and allow time for the person to sort things out for himself before redefining how you can love one another.

- Be willing to be used. Often when we say, "I feel used!" we mean that we feel taken advantage of. When it comes to helping a loved one who has cancer, being useful is a great privilege, and you can make yourself available in many ways. The best way to help is by offering specific, concrete assistance with the kinds of tasks that the ill person cannot do for himself at that time. For example, friends can help a lot by offering to bring over dinner on Friday night. Be sure to ask about dietary restrictions and the preferences of the patient and family, set a definite time to drop off the food, and *leave*. It is a special treat to eat food lovingly prepared just for you when it is hot and at its most appetizing. You don't do much of a favor if you intrude on the dinner hour.

Another common need for those with cancer, especially those who usually do the household chores, is help with housework. Ask if you can come while the patient is at treatment and wash the kitchen floor, dust the living room, change the sheets, wash the bedroom windows or do the laundry. Cancer takes a lot of time. Even if the patient isn't the homemaker, priorities have shifted and extra help is often welcome. Consider offering help with outside chores: Prune the roses, rake the leaves, shovel the snow, or take the car for servicing. Be creative. The gift of your time and energy will be deeply appreciated.

- Walk along on the journey. Obviously this depends on how close you are to the patient and on your own availability. Some of the most profoundly helpful times for me occurred when a friend just sat with me and silently held my hand. Having a support person along for doctor's appointments or treatments can be nurturing. Remember that you are the *support* person and be sure not to intrude on the problem-solving that is strictly between the patient and physician. Sometimes as a support person you may be invited by the patient to express concerns or negative emotions. For example, you might be asked to say, "My wife was upset by your statement last visit that you thought she might need additional chemotherapy. What exactly did you mean by that comment?" *Only* speak on behalf of the patient if you have his or her express permission to do so. Remember that you are there as an invited guest and that the patient or the physician may need to ask you to leave at any time.

- Validate feelings. Be willing to recognize and accept both the happy, optimistic feelings and the discouraged ones. The patient has a right to be negative, withdrawn or silent and that does not mean that she has given up or has a bad attitude. It is much more helpful to say, "I see you are feeling discouraged today" than to say, "Cheer up!" If she could, she would! Recognize that up and down days are normal.

- Use touch to reassure and express your love and support. When a person is feeling ill, they often have a hunger for being held and consoled. Sometimes the best help for the pain, inner and outer, is a long, very gentle hug. Another way to express the same caring is through a gentle backrub or foot massage. The goal isn't to relax tense muscles, although that may happen, but to speak your support with body language. Be tender. Be prepared for tears during this time. Allowing someone to weep safely with you is an important way you can help him restore his emotional balance.

- If you are a person of faith, ask permission to pray for the patient, then do it consistently and regularly as a promise to be kept. The prayers of friends and relatives can surround a patient with peace through even the most demanding physical challenges. Not only will the patient feel the results, but you will find that simply calling his needs to mind on a daily basis will remind you of other ways to help. Prayer may trigger your memory to buy and send a card or to make an extra effort to keep in touch. When you see the patient, you might ask if she has a particular prayer intention, then pray specifically for that. The emotional and spiritual challenges of cancer are often the most troubling, and knowing that prayers are being offered can be tremendously reassuring. I remember praying, "God, look at all these people who are praying for me. You wouldn't want to disappoint all of them, would you?"

- Make a commitment to yourself—and share it with the patient—that you will be available as a friend and support person for the long haul. At the beginning of the cancer journey it seems the mailbox is full of good wishes every day and your home is full of bouquets and plants. Sadly some friends respond once and then seem to think they have done their duty. They move on to other matters, figuring the patient knows, of course, that they care. Actually the cards, phone calls, and visits are even more precious after three or six months of treatment when it seems as if the whole world has gone back to normal. The patient is still ill and may feel forgotten, as well. Make a promise to yourself and your loved one that you will not lose interest. Pledge to love her even if her hair falls out. Promise to be there if he is queasy from chemotherapy. Reach out and touch her even if she looks "terrible." For the patient, fear of abandonment can be as scary as the fear of the disease. The most important gift you may be able to give is the assurance that he will never be so sick that you will stop loving him. Even if visits can last only a few minutes, those few minutes may be the most important time in the day for someone who is critically ill. Don't worry about what you will say, simply be there and be willing to express your love.

- Say "Call anytime" and mean it. The darkest hours are often in the middle of the night, and a friend then is a treasure beyond compare.

In short:

- Don't tell horror stories or any anecdote that adds to fear or apprehension.

- Don't throw out advice.

- Don't say, "I know how you feel."

- Don't pry or be nosy.

- Don't avoid your friend because you are unsure what to say or do.

- Do be available but not intrusive.

- Do ask before you drop in for a visit and let the patient set the time and length of stay.

- Do be willing to be used in whatever way the patient needs help.

- Do share the journey.

- Do use touch to express your care and support.

- Do ask permission to pray for the patient and follow through.

- Do make a commitment to yourself and your friend that you will not abandon him or her.

- Do respect privacy and confidentiality.

- Do validate feelings. "It's hard! You're tired!"

Social Issues

And let your best be for your friend,
If he must know the ebb of your tide,
Let him know its flood also.
(Kahlil Gibran, *The Prophet*)

Isolation or loneliness can make the cancer journey much more difficult. Sadly a few friends or even family members will draw away from you with comments such as, "I just can't bring myself to go see her. It is too hard for me. I have never been good around sick people. What would I say?" Their own fears can paralyze them or blind them to your need and the chance for them to learn and grow. Sometimes, as they get used to the idea that you are still the same person they have known and loved and that you just happen to have cancer now, they will tentatively begin to approach you, usually with an impersonal card or a safe phone call. Since you are the person who needs all the support you can get right now, it makes sense to encourage your friends and family to help in the ways you prefer. Many people will say, "I just don't know what to do," and so they do nothing. It may feel awkward to ask for assistance if you are a person who is accustomed to *giving* help or support. Put yourself in the shoes of your friend. If someone asked you for help, would you be put off or delighted to know what you could do? Give your friends the benefit of the doubt. Don't let fears of "How will I ever repay them?" keep you from giving your friends the gift of participating in your journey. Love isn't about repayment but about receiving love from one and passing it on to another, according to the seasons of our lives.

How can well-wishers help? Driving carpools (or you to appointments), making meals, doing laundry, cleaning house, paying bills, writing letters, praying, or just sitting quietly with you may all be welcome at different times. One of the nicest gifts I received during my illness was a gift of song. A teenager had done a beautiful solo presentation at our church, and I asked her mother for a copy of the words because they touched my heart. The mom and daughter decided to make a tape recording for me, but when the tape recorder jammed, the daughter suggested that she come and sing the song for me in person before she left for college. The mother was amazed at the suggestion, but called and asked if they could come over. I will never forget how loved I felt receiving this unexpected gift of self and talent from a shy eighteen-year-old.

At my four-day checkup after my mastectomy I was told that my particular health history and tumor type required a second mastectomy before I could begin chemotherapy. The doctors suggested a surgery date three days away. I was stunned, weak, scared, and sure I would have an emotional breakdown if I followed that advice. Knowing that my husband's job commitments could not be abandoned at such short notice, I told him, "The only way I can possibly go through with this surgery is if I can count on "babysitters" for the next three weeks. If I have a dear, trusted friend with me for three hours each morning and three hours each afternoon, I think I can make it." I was too distraught to make the calls, so I compiled a list of people who would be appropriate companions and asked a good friend to call and set up a schedule. My requirements were quite stringent. My "helpers" needed to be people with whom I felt comfortable enough that I would not need to put on a show or be a hostess. They needed to be forewarned that during those three hours their *only* agenda was to support me in whatever way I needed support. My visitors needed to be prepared that they could find me without makeup or in bed. I might be sleepy or weepy. I might want to talk or just be quiet. Perhaps I would need a ride somewhere, or I might want a walking companion. I might be reasonable or unreasonable. Their only job was to provide a loving presence for me.

The results of this desperate reaching out were quite amazing. My scheduler was able to put together a calendar as I had requested. These were all busy people, and I felt awful asking for their time. I knew they would have to rearrange their own needs to meet mine. When I voiced my concern, my buddy said, "Do you have any idea how happy these people are to help you? Every one of them was delighted to be asked and to know how they could help you through such a hard time. They felt it was an honor to be able to do this."

As it turned out, I had a wonderful time during that recovery period. The friendships that had been barely glowing (too busy) were fanned into full flame again. We laughed together, cried, and grew closer through our shared challenges. We caught up on all the old news. I came to the end of the three weeks not only strong enough to cope on my own but filled with joy at the pleasure of being with friends. I felt so good, in fact, that I made a vow to plan at least one date with a friend every week to keep the relationships healthy and to treat us both.

Sometimes the social problem you have to deal with is not too few friends but too many. This can be equally distressing. While you are in the hospital you cannot use your time to recover if you are up all night and "entertaining" all day. How do you set limits?

A good way to keep everyone informed and still preserve your sanity is to designate a telephone contact person outside of your own household—maybe a close friend, a neighbor, or a family member. After surgery, anyone wanting to express good wishes or get an update can call for the latest news without disturbing you. It can be draining for the patient to tell the same story over and over again. This contact person can also relay requests for help to your friends—for example, to arrange a carpool ride for a child or to bring over dinner on Tuesday. In this age of instant contact through Facebook and other social media, you may be able to use the Internet to your advantage. An excellent resource is CaringBridge. com, a free service that lets you stay in contact with those people you choose. You post updates and receive replies at your convenience.

Another alternative is to enlist the help of the hospital staff. At the time of my second mastectomy, I asked that a "no visitors" sign be posted on my door. Right then I was so emotionally raw that I did not want to talk to anyone, and my concern with being nice or appreciative was far less important than self-preservation.

At home, my answering machine recorded good wishes, which I loved, and allowed me to decide at the moment of the call if talking to a particular person would make me feel better or worse. We all have friends who can be counted on to cheer us up. Other friends routinely require more energy than they give. It is perfectly all right to choose the timing of calls to suit your needs. I chose to return certain calls the next morning, when I would be at my most rested, alert, and positive, and to answer other calls immediately.

Be bold. Be creative. Take the initiative by making a phone call, sending a note, saying hi on the street. No matter how you are feeling, be a person your friends want to be with. You can be honest about your occasional down times if you also are willing to share the up times. If you don't allow others to be close to you, everyone loses.

A final note. A handful of my friends have silently slipped away, their fears too great or their courage and compassion too small to risk contact. I am saddened by this, but I take comfort in the fact that they were invited to grow and chose to remain in their safe, healthy world. Their choice is out of my control. *My* choice is to give and receive love.

In short:

- Try to maintain friendships by being the kind of person others want to be with.

- Allow others to help with food, rides, or yard needs.

- If you are overwhelmed with visits or calls, use an answering machine or voice mail to screen calls, put up a "no visitors" sign at the hospital, or designate a phone update person who is not in your household.

- Take the initiative to call or write to stay in touch through the long days of treatment.

The Soul Perspective

I almost didn't include this chapter because I was afraid of losing readers who deal with their spirituality in a way different from me. My reasons to include it were twofold. First, my spiritual life is the most important single factor in my survival, both physical and emotional, through this cancer journey. The second consideration was that since this is a "choose your own adventure" type book, no one is a captive audience. Because God was such an integral part of my recovery, I intend to be honest about the spiritual components of wellness for me. For you who want to rediscover or renew your own faith, read on.

As a young adult, for my entire life before cancer, I found myself putting spiritual issues on a back burner. I thought I would deal with them later because right now I was too busy and I felt inadequate to answer the tough questions. They seemed too scary and too complicated. I planned to consider the big questions sometime when I was fresh, alert, uninterrupted, and calm. Guess what—I pushed them aside all my adult life. The time was never right.

My questions included: What do I believe about God? How do I understand creation? What do I think happens after I die? What do I have to show for my life's work?

How can I continue to affect my loved ones through the dying process and after my death? Obviously these issues are the core of who we are as human beings. I have often described my diagnosis of ovarian cancer as the equivalent of a sledgehammer blow to the head from God. Suddenly "later" was right now, the questions were inescapable, and they often kept me awake at night.

I had had a variety of minor health problems in my recent past, including mononucleosis at age forty. I knew that I was not living a balanced or healthy life that respected the needs of my body. I was skimping on sleep, grabbing fast food and wolfing it down, racing from one activity to the next in a state of constant turmoil, trying to pack one more activity into each frenzied day. The minor health problems were taps on the shoulder, which should have gotten my attention and led me to change my ways. My cancer diagnosis led me to the immediate response, "OK, God. You have my full attention now. I'm listening!" I came to a firm determination that I would never live that harried existence again. (I don't believe that God caused my cancer, but I do believe he used this natural event to bring me blessings.)

As I prayed for guidance, it became clear to me at each step of the way what I should do. My goal was to be obedient to God and to get back on track to live as a faith-filled, joy-filled person. In my response to the overwhelming demands of things to do, I had lost sight of the big picture, of the "why" that is so important. Instead of being faith-filled and joy-filled, I was full of frustration and anxiety. My first step was simple: Put aside everything that took time and attention away from my health. I spent a week resigning from every activity and outside commitment. It was painful to give up the leadership of a Girl Scout troop and the board of the Youth Chorus. I didn't want to stop working in my children's classrooms. I hated to disappoint all those who were counting on me to prepare presentations or organize fund-raisers. It was absolutely clear to me, however, that unless I gave my full attention to wellness, I was never going to be well. My daily planner, so chock-full of commitments that I would run out of room to record appointments, was symbolically relegated to a bottom drawer of my dresser for the first several weeks after my surgery. (It did come out after that, but it was filled with doctors' appointments and yoga classes instead of "should's.") My "to do" list became only a memory-jogger, so that when I had some free time I might consider how I chose to fill it. It had previously been "marching orders" for the day, week and month—with no end in sight. (Just a note—as I returned to health, I was able and delighted to resume some of the important work I loved but with care and attention to my overall well-being.)

Interestingly enough, two close friends about my age in our church had been diagnosed with life-threatening illnesses just before I was. Their families chose to be open and honest about the diagnosis. They spoke clearly and freely about desperately wanting and needing prayer. I knew from my own experience the joy and sense of participation that comes from praying for a friend in need, and this lesson served me well. I was able to ask for help right from the start, for the precious help that comes from knowing you are prayed for. Each person who offered to help received the same request, "Please pray for me." These prayers were my lifeline during procedures that were too scary to face any other way. I absolutely could feel the grace and protection from fear that resulted from being "covered in prayer." In fact, the prayers had such a dramatic impact on me that at one point I asked my spiritual advisor, "What will happen to me if these people stop praying?" He answered that that was God's business, not mine. God would bring me to the minds of these friends as I needed the prayers. Experience showed this to be true. An added advantage was that everyone who wanted to help could. I could begin every conversation with an expression of thanks for prayers instead of a litany of complaints or a recital of aches and pains.

One of the greatest sources of consolation and healing for me came through the sacraments in my church. The Anointing of the Sick is a prayer and blessing for those who are seriously ill. I was blessed to receive this sacrament before my surgeries, and the prayers for healing were surely answered, not only in my physical recovery but even more by the change in my spiritual life. If your church offers any such opportunity for community prayer, take advantage of it!

Another source of help and hope came from a wide variety of books available, both for those on the cancer journey and for those who simply want to find direction for their life, healthy or sick. I can't mention every book that shaped my thought, but the first book I received as a gift, *Love, Medicine, and Miracles* by Bernie Siegel, was a powerful introduction to the new life I was facing. I continue to recommend this book to everyone newly diagnosed with cancer. In addition, many books exploring the spiritual dimensions of the healing process lifted my spirits and redirected my energies. *The Road Less Traveled* by M. Scott Peck is a classic, and it outlines a framework for avoiding self-pity and growing through adversity, which is the human condition! Take some time to explore your local library or bookstore and check the bibliography for resources that will lift *your* spirit.

I am fortunate, too, to meet on a weekly basis with a group of Christian women who pray, study the Bible, and share our faith journeys. This group became (and still is) my support group as I returned to health. My commitment to the Tuesday morning Bible study was the first thing entered in my date book for the week, and the ongoing focus it provided was a huge help to avoid the pitfalls of isolation and feeling sorry for myself.

I was baptized Catholic as an infant and learned from the time I was a child that suffering has a purpose and has meaning in its own right. I remember as a student in Catholic school being told to "offer it up" when problems came my way. This concept includes the desire to help others, the awareness that suffering is not random or simply negative, and the willingness to approach one's own suffering with the attitude that pain can be used by God for good. It is apparent even from secular psychology how my pain can help *me* grow. In addition, I believe that my prayer, fasting, and good works can help *others,* or why would I pray? If that is so, my decision to make my acceptance of suffering a gift to God on behalf of someone else is a form of active prayer. While I was ill, so many others faced much greater pain—the loss of a child, mental illness, the death of a spouse—that I never had a shortage of those who needed prayer. During some of the hardest hours, I was able to bear my own misery with a more peaceful heart because I named and prayed for a specific person who needed God's grace and peace right at that moment. None of us will ever know how much our actions and intentions influence others. What is clear is that my choice blessed *me* and gave meaning to experiences that were very difficult. I believe my suffering, offered for others, helped them in ways that can't be quantified.

One barrier to a full-hearted participation in faith for me was my scientific background. I have a degree in biology and have worked in a medical laboratory. I was trained to see disease as a set of causes and effects that could be entirely explained by the scientific method. Treatment of illness became an exercise in choosing the correct drug or surgery. My instinct to explain still remains, but I am learning that science is only one approach to the mystery of our life.

During my treatment, I attended a lecture at Santa Clara University by a professor, a Jesuit priest, who spoke on "mythical reality." It was the best explanation I have ever heard of the dilemma of conflict between science and spirituality.

He described two different realities, both of which are truth. In Western culture we have grown accustomed to thinking that only scientific reality can be true. In other words, if you can't see it, measure it, touch it, poke it, or explain it, then it can't be truth. He said that the scientific approach is only one way to see reality. A different reality exists simultaneously with the scientific one. Scientific truth compares finite data with finite observations. Mythic truth, on the other hand, deals with the infinite. Some people call this truth spiritual. This kind of truth requires you to participate in the observation and draw meaning from it. It includes real things like the love of a parent for a child and the unmeasurable but certain knowledge of the heart that God exists. Just because it can't be proved doesn't mean that it is not real. He said that the reason it cannot be proved is because it is beyond the usual parameters of our senses and requires the knowledge of our heart. I believe the ideas of Eastern religion and medicine about the energy forces in the body fall into this category, as does the power of the mind in the healing of the body (see bibliography, *The Anatomy of Hope* and *Radical Remission*). Many other truths are also beyond explanation.

As I began to take stock of my spiritual status during the early stages of my illness, I experienced "the fear of the Lord" when I considered the state of my soul. I was shocked to realize that I actually acted and believed at a deep level that I was as good as God, that I knew as much as God, and that I really didn't need God much except for emergencies. I pretty much thought I could handle just about anything that came my way on my own. It was profoundly humbling to have my self-importance restored to its rightful place: God as the creator, me as his created child. Like the prodigal son, I found myself returning to God with remorse and sorrow. In time, after several days, I began to believe that I was forgiven and to thank God for giving me a second chance. I resolved to change both my actions and my priorities. This insight was a turning point in my search for peace.

Another erroneous attitude was my belief that if I only could try harder and "be better" I would be free of problems and be in control not just of me, but of my husband, my children, and everyone else! I was convinced that if I did everything right I would have perfectly behaved children, good health, a happy marriage, and no problems. I have no idea where I formed this world view, but it is amazing how different everything looks to me now. I came to realize that like all human beings, I will die. As the author William Saroyan put it, "I always knew that people don't live forever, but somehow in my case I thought there would be an exception made." God will not make an exception in my case! I also realized that I have no ability to direct the really fundamental needs of my life, such as my heartbeat or next breath. I am not in control! My own efforts can never bring me the power that belongs only to God. When I accepted my own limitations, I opened up space in my consciousness to perceive the action of God. It had been there all along, only I couldn't see it.

How do I see God acting in my life? I can give examples, but in the final analysis faith is required to see these events as God's work. The first experience was a result of the profound shock of looking death in the face. It was such an overwhelming time for me that I could do nothing to escape the constant awareness that I could die at any moment. I remember standing in my room in the grand hotel in Yosemite National Park and breaking into sobs because I might never be able to return to that beautiful place. Even watching a video or reading the newspaper became difficult for me because I didn't want to "waste" any time that could be used to express my love to my family and friends. My state of mind was similar to depression but with a different emphasis. I was not sad but rather keenly aware of the passing of time and the constant opportunity and responsibility of using time wisely. This intense perception lasted for many weeks and finally was transformed in a moment's insight. I saw that I was alive at that moment and that all I could do was to live in that place, for that time. I actually said, "I'm not dead yet!" This change of perspective came from God and freed me to function in the day-to-day world with some level of normalcy.

The second experience I had of God's comforting touch came through the amazing timing of encouraging and uplifting gestures of other people. It was uncanny how just when I needed a lift the phone would ring and a buddy would say, "I'm thinking of you. I love you." Or the mail would bring a card from a longtime friend, just to cheer me. Or a stranger would stop (bald) me on the street and say, "Last year I had no hair. I am fine now. I just wanted you to know that people do recover." Time after time the medical personnel caring for me would reassure me and reach out in especially loving ways. I still have the gift I received from my infusion nurse as a celebration of the end of my chemo treatments. I know these people are good-hearted, but I believe that God gave them a nudge to reach out to me exactly when I needed the most encouragement.

I also felt a keen sense of God's peace around me as I faced some of the most difficult procedures. While I was having my first CT scan, I was actually shaking with fear. I asked the tech if it would interfere with the results if I was trembling. It would. I turned to God. One breath at a time, I prayed the name "Jesus" over and over, for a very long thirty minutes. I felt a soft cocoon of peace surround me, invisible but warm and comforting, protecting me from harm. This peace was definitely a gift to me, not something that I could make happen on my own. It got me through some painful and very scary times. God's hand was in it. I could feel my prayers and the prayers of my friends being answered.

One of the most beautiful touches of God came on a gray morning when I was feeling especially overwhelmed and depressed. My cancer seemed to be so strong, so relentless, and I felt so vulnerable. I was struggling with little effect to lift my spirits. As I walked into my bathroom, I caught my breath at the sight of a sunbeam that found its way through the pulled curtains. It fell on a single, perfect iris bloom that

I had picked the day before. I can still see that exquisite purple flower, spotlighted by the sun. When I looked, I could see the fine detail in the petals, almost as if I could see the translucent, glistening cells that together formed this perfect whole. I marveled at the wonder of God, who could knit together chemicals and compounds to make such a beautiful flower. And with a flood of comfort I realized that the same God who made that flower and ordered those cells to combine had the power and love to order the cells in my body to be made whole.

Besides being a source of comfort and peace, God continues to provide direction for my actions. I stopped asking myself, "What can I do here?" and started asking, "What is God's will for me to do in this situation?" I feel an urgency to use the time I have been given wisely. I don't waste time. Even my reading habits have changed. If the book I am reading does not touch me, I don't hesitate to put it aside, no matter how many people have recommended it. Before cancer, I felt obligated to "finish what I started." The opinion of other people is much less important to me and the eternal measure of my actions is a far greater concern. For several months my job description was to be a "freelance lover," to keep my eyes open for those who were suffering and to reach out my hand in companionship and friendship. I have learned to be keenly aware of my own limits. I still filter my immediate impulses through the question, "Can I do this good thing without compromising my own needs for rest, exercise, and emotional strength?" I am convinced that God will not call me to act in a way that disregards my health needs. The guidance, which I felt so strongly during my cancer journey, continues.

God's long-term work for me unfolds day by day. On one of my walks, when I was just starting to have some extra energy after my chemotherapy, I was musing about the future. I casually asked God if He had any ideas for the rest of my life, this great and thrilling gift of time and health. To my astonishment, immediately the thought came to me, "I want you to be example." Talk about scary! My immediate reaction was, "I'd rather write a book!" Being example meant that I would have to live in a way that other cancer patients could learn from and desire for themselves. I would have to continue to be committed to taking good care of myself if I was encouraging others to do so. I would have to be vulnerable enough to share my story with people who might misunderstand or ridicule me. It might even mean that I would have to undergo more "adventures" with cancer. I slowly and tentatively began to live according to this directive. I make conscious, sometimes daily, decisions to encourage those struggling with cancer. I accompany friends to doctors' appointments. I listen, I write notes, I pray. To my surprise this giving gives to me most of all—my life is full of meaning and joy.

Life remains for me a sweet, unexpected surprise. I begin each day with a prayer of thanks to God for the incomprehensible privilege of being alive. I savor the times with my grandchildren, children, husband and friends. Each family gathering brings the thought, "I might never have been here! Isn't God good?" I am much more willing to set aside my own agenda when an opportunity comes my way to express my love, whether it is going to a movie with my family or helping out an elderly friend. I enjoy the chance to travel across town or across the ocean. I walk through each day marveling at the beauty that surrounds me.

When I was unsure if I would survive my adventure with cancer, I made a promise, "If I am healed, I will give God all the honor and glory." This book is one way I attempt to do that.

In short:

- Acknowledge that God is in control of your life and circumstances.

- Pray for guidance about decisions along the way.

- Be open enough to ask your faith community to pray for you.

- Receive the prayers of elders or the sacraments if they are available to you.

- Read inspirational books and short stories about people who have found joy in spite of their problems.

- Join or start a faith support group, such as a weekly Bible study.

- Remember that there is a great deal of reality that science can't explain and believe that God works in ways beyond our understanding.

- Seek God's will for your use of time and talents as you continue treatments and return to health.
- Give thanks!

A New (Healthy) Beginning

The beginning of cancer treatment is an excellent time to change habits, build new routines, and nurture your body as much as possible. Consider yourself in training, as if you are an athlete preparing for a competition. How can you do this? Each person's path to wellness is different, but the questions to consider apply to all of us.

- How much sleep do you need to feel your best? Do you feel better if you sleep all at once at night or if you nap once or twice a day? Try it out. Explore your options.

- What kind of food fills you with vitality? What makes you sluggish? When are the best times for you to eat? Sometimes breakfast was my main meal of the day. That's OK!

- Are you eating a well-balanced diet? If your food intake is unpredictable, ask your doctor about the possibility of adding a pre-natal vitamin daily to protect you from deficiency.

- Are your immunizations up to date? Ask your doctor about flu shots, pneumonia vaccine, and shingles vaccination.

- How much exercise do you need? What kind of exercise appeals to you, and how often?

- What people nurture you? Who is a good listener, an unconditionally loving friend? How can you be in touch with him or her? Phone calls, letters, a cup of tea, text messages, a visit between rounds of chemo?

- What spiritual practice makes you feel integrated? Daily prayer, meditation, Bible study, inspirational books, and religious services are all options. What do *you* need?

- What activities or services bring meaning to your life, lift you up and give you joy? Maybe driving the carpool is a precious and meaningful way to stay connected to your children and their lives. Perhaps you love to write or paint, garden or play golf. If you find yourself confined to a job or a set of tasks that drains you, honestly consider whether you can allow yourself to take sick leave to set aside time for your healing. If your job brings you joy, then continuing it may be your best path. In any case, the key is to examine the components of your life and decide anew what to keep and what to let go. Ideally the decision is based on a simple question: Does this activity feed me, lift me up, make me feel better and more alive? Or does it drain me, tire me, or make me feel worse? Choose life!

- What is play for you? Reading a good book, getting together with friends, playing a musical instrument, gathering seashells? Let your imagination live again, and consider how you can build a "play time" into your schedule.

- How can you focus on health rather than illness? I found myself worrying about forgetting to take my medications. Sometimes I was unable to remember if I had taken them that day. I purchased daily pill containers at the pharmacy. Each holds a week's worth of medicine. I use one for the morning medications and one for the evening ones. I juggle all the pill bottles once every three weeks instead of twice a day. I can tell at a glance if I have taken my medications for that day. Cutting down on the time and emphasis spent on pills and how sick I am allows me to focus instead on how good I am feeling.

- What are the sources of stress in your life? Can you take action now to reduce that stress? Something as simple as updating your will can be a source of relief. Putting your affairs in order doesn't have to be ominous: It simply frees you from worry. Many hospitals provide information on durable power of attorney for health care and your wishes for your care if you are unable to communicate. An excellent document that provides the legal directives with heart is *Five Wishes* (see bibliography). Take the time to think about your choices and put them in writing. You can then proceed with your care knowing you have done everything possible to clarify your wishes for your providers and your family.

- Look for *progress* in regaining health, rather than setting an impossible immediate goal: I want to be back to normal! Goals should be measurable and attainable. If they are too hard to achieve, you may be tempted to give up. For example, try to walk a little further, even a few more steps, each day. Do one more repetition of a stretching exercise each day. Just for today, choose some carrots instead of a piece of candy. Over time you will see the cumulative effect of increasing fitness.

Once you have chosen the components of a healthy life for you, give yourself permission to set up a schedule that nurtures you. If at all possible, let this treatment time be a time when your own health is your top priority. I realize that responsibilities press in on us all. A job or caring for others (children, parents, sibling, or spouse) may be necessary. But you can decide to use your discretionary time to increase your health instead of sitting mindlessly in front of the TV or computer or stressing out over details of things to do. When the demands of daily life crowded in on me, I would ask, "What would happen if I choose not to do the laundry today?" The world did not stop. Often one hour or one day's delay doesn't matter, and I found myself living in incredible freedom from the "should's" of life. Most of us are our own worst taskmasters.

As I began my cancer journey, I wrote out a constitution for myself, incorporating the healthy habits I knew were important for me. Putting my decisions down in writing and posting them on my mirror gave me a constant reminder that I was building *new* habits, not just drifting along as usual.

Another helpful coping technique is to keep a diary recording how you feel on an hour-by-hour or day-by-day basis. This way you can discover patterns. For example, you may find that chemo day three, for you, is a day when you feel depressed, but day four and five are up days as your energy returns. The next cycle, on day three, you can be reassured that better days are ahead.

Even after you are doing all you can do, you may be troubled by side effects such as fatigue, nausea, loss of appetite, changes in skin or hair or nails, or a general feeling of ill health. It can be helpful to check out the American Cancer Society's materials for suggestions about specific strategies to try. For example, you can learn what kinds of food are most easily tolerated (see bibliography, *Eating Well Through Cancer*). Talking to someone who has been there can be a great help. Often non-medical tips (the use of a hot water bottle, a back rub, or a hot bath) have helped someone else cope and may also help you. Even if you do not find relief from your symptoms, you will probably feel better just talking to someone who understands!

In short:

• Inventory your own personal "good health" needs for

sleep, food, social contact, spiritual practice, and work-related activities.

- Consider how to include play in your life.

- Focus on health, not illness.

- Look for *progress* in regaining health. Don't wait for the long-term goal of "returning to normal."

- Draw up a schedule or a contract with yourself to incorporate health needs into your day.

- Keep a diary to trigger your memory about what works and what does not.

Logistics—Who, What, Where, When?

⚜

It used to be so easy. You got sick, you went to your family doctor (who delivered your children and gave you all your shots) and he made you better. What does a thinking person do about medical care in the 21st century? This chapter can't tell you what to do, unfortunately, but it can suggest the questions you might want to consider as you set out to treat and hopefully cure your cancer.

Who provides the care is a critical question. In many cases, the "who" will determine the rest of your choices. A physician confirms your cancer diagnosis, usually based on results from a biopsy. Your next step is to ask that doctor for his or her recommendations for surgeons, radiation oncologists, and/or medical oncologists. In some cases your local doctors may be among the best trained, best equipped, and most up-to-date in the country. This obviously depends on where you live. In other cases, especially if you are in a remote or rural area, the care you need may not even be available locally, and you will need to travel regardless of your preferences. One way to evaluate the expertise of your doctors is to ask if they are board certified in their specialty.

Board-certified doctors have not only completed extra training, but they have also passed a rigorous exam. What choice will you make if your local doctors are pretty good but your child or spouse is urging you to go to the "top cancer doctor" in the country?

Your decision needs to take several variables into account. First of all, is your cancer a commonly seen, uncomplicated one? If so, the advice you receive may well be the same at a major cancer center as at your local surgeon's office. If you have a cancer that is unusual because it is rare, especially aggressive, or in an area of the body that is hard to reach, you may want to get an opinion at a cancer center. Doctors at these regional centers see more cases of cancer similar to yours and usually have more experience dealing with complicated treatments. One difficulty with going to a cancer center is that your appointment may be days or weeks away, and you may be anxious to "get on with it." Understandably, time delays cause additional worry. This is a major decision, however, and you will live with the consequences for the rest of your life. Usually a delay of up to two weeks will not put you at significantly greater risk. That time to check out your options may result in peace of mind for you and be worth the wait.

The second thing to consider is your support system. If you travel to a distant city or state for your treatments, how will this impact your overall wellness? At home, you know who to call for moral support, assistance with housekeeping chores, or emergency car repairs. In a distant city or state your support may be limited to the staff at the cancer center. Usually these employees are excellent at reassuring people away from home, but they will not know you the way your hometown support people do. Your contact with family and friends may be limited to phone calls and emails instead of daily hugs and visits. How will that affect you?

Thirdly, you will want to consider the extra stress of organizing your responsibilities from a distance. You still will have bills to pay, pets to feed, and lawns to mow whether you are home or not. Do you have a friend or family member who can stay in your house or step in and take care of the logistics of running your home in your absence?

Often a cancer center can establish a treatment plan that can be administered in your own area. You may be able to receive chemotherapy or radiation treatments locally, based on the decisions made by out-of-town experts at a cancer center. Whatever decision you make about who your doctors will be, you can still seek second or even third opinions during the course of your treatment.

What kind of treatment is best for you? You might think this is a clear-cut question, but in fact often several options are supported by research and current practice. For example, it is not unusual for highly competent oncologists to differ in their recommendations for a chemotherapy drug. It isn't a matter of right versus wrong but of benefits versus risks. Like anyone else, a doctor may be conservative or liberal by nature or by training. Differing recommendations can be confusing to you, but it is still important to know what the choices are before you agree to a treatment plan. In today's world of medicine, your treatment will often be established based on the recommendations of a team of doctors, and you are a part of the team, too. Your personal lifestyle, risk tolerance, and body image concerns need to be included as a part of the decision.

When will your treatments begin? Sometimes an emergency problem such as a bowel obstruction requires immediate surgery, and the discussion must wait. Often, though, you will have a few days or even weeks to gather information, have additional diagnostic tests, and then decide on the best course of action. You may be tempted to avoid making the decision by procrastinating. There is a tendency to do so much research that you become hopelessly bogged down with details you don't understand. You can become paralyzed with indecision. It is critical to set yourself a deadline for making your decision and stick to it so that important care will not be postponed indefinitely.

Before the actual doctor's visit, write down a list of your questions. Leave space after the questions to jot down the answers. It is hard to concentrate without a memory jogger. The medical name of your tumor will be used to determine all of the treatment choices, so it is good to have it written down for your reference. It will help you to know if your tumor is rare or is the form of breast, prostate or lung cancer most commonly seen. Treatment will depend on the size of the tumor and the involvement of surrounding tissues and/ or lymph nodes. Often this information is not available at the time of diagnosis—from a biopsy, for instance—but if it is known, ask for it. You might want to see an anatomical chart or sketch showing exactly where your tumor is. Ask what kinds of treatment are most effective for your cancer type—surgery? radiation? chemotherapy? If more than one kind of treatment is recommended, in what order are they given? Ask how you can expect to feel after the treatment and how long you should expect for recovery. Even though each person's response varies, you will want to know, for instance, if you will not be able to drive for two weeks. For your own reassurance, you might want to ask your doctor about how many patients with your kind of cancer he or she treats in a year.

The most important question to ask is the one that frightens you the most, whatever that is. Maybe it is whether you will lose your hair, or be nauseated, or be unable to have children, or have a big scar. Whatever is tops on *your* list, *ask*. You will then have additional time to start dealing with the emotional challenges before you are feeling bad from surgery or chemotherapy. And you might find out that this concern does not apply in your case!

What not to ask? "How long do I have to live?" "What are my chances of a cure?" No one can give you these answers. It is far more helpful to you to know ways to increase your wellness during treatment and to strengthen your body than to be depressed by statistics, which are really meaningless in an individual case. If your cancer is cured, the cure rate is 100 percent for you!

In short:

- Take the time you need—and set yourself a time limit—to evaluate your options in terms of medical care providers, location of facility, and type of care provided.

- Ask prospective doctors if they are board-certified and how many cases similar to yours they treat in a year.

- As you make your decisions, include factors such as the type of cancer, the availability of support systems, the cost and stress of travel, and the logistics of running a home or job.

- Ask questions about both the benefits and risks of different treatment approaches so you can make the decision that you believe is best for you.

- Be sure to write down both questions and answers so you can remember what was said. This is true throughout treatment.

- The most important question is the one that scares you the most. You may discover that you have been worrying needlessly about something that will not even be an issue for you.

Being a Good Patient: Your Place on the Team

The days are gone when doctors were gods and patients were treated as if they were children. Today's more highly educated patients expect to be treated as the adults they are. In fact, every patient is protected by a "Patient's Bill of Rights." You can request a copy of this from your doctor or hospital. In summary, it states that you are entitled to respect, information, and competent care.

Along with these rights, every patient also has responsibilities to self and to the care providers. It is your responsibility to ask questions if you don't understand. Sometimes it can feel awkward to interrupt a long explanation about your care. You want to be polite, so you think you'll save your questions till the end. While you are making a mental note about your question, you miss the next point. Then another question comes up, and you lose the first one entirely. At the end of the explanation when you are asked, "Any questions?" you have forgotten them. To avoid this, use a visual cue. As soon as you don't understand something, hold up your hand as a stop sign. Politely say, "I'm sorry, I didn't catch that." You can ask for the information to be repeated or explained in a different way. You can ask how to spell a medical term (take notes). You can ask related questions, such as "What happens after that?" At the end of the explanation you want to be able to say you *do* understand. Your doctor wants this, too.

Two additional patient responsibilities are important. You agree to treat your caregivers with respect (including the janitor who empties your trash can). It is your job to cooperate with the recommendations of your doctors or to discuss with them why you are not willing to do so.

The head of your traditional (orthodox) healing team will be your oncologist. He or she may be an M.D. (medical doctor) or a D.O. (doctor of osteopathy). Both of these professionals go through a rigorous training program and are equally well-prepared to provide your care. Doctors of osteopathy have an additional focus on the possibilities of manipulating muscles and bones to increase structural integrity. Non-physician health-care providers support the doctors. These include the Nurse Practitioner, N.P., who is a registered nurse with an advanced degree in nursing practice studies. The N.P. can provide care independently or in collaboration with a physician. The Physician's Assistant, P.A., has a bachelor's degree and has completed an additional thirty-three months of training. Both N.P.s and P.A.s work under the supervision of a physician but may make independent medical decisions, too. The registered nurse, R.N., has completed rigorous training in the clinical part of the job and is often the direct provider of care in an office or hospital setting (giving infusions, for example). Other care-providers include L.V.N.s, who provide for the non-medical needs of patients such as bathing or toileting and are under the direction of doctors and R.N.s; Physical Therapists, P.T.s, who assist with strengthening the body; Occupational Therapists, O.T.s, who are excellent for adapting your routines and assistive tools to the new needs of your body; and a wide range of other specialized therapists. As a patient, you have the daunting task of keeping all of these people straight. If you are unsure, it is always OK to ask someone, "Who are you?" Often P.A.s and N.P.s will be your first contact, and they will refer you to a doctor if necessary. Give them a chance. Don't demand to see the doctor unless you have a concern that is not met by them.

Your care will involve interactions with dozens of providers from nurses to lab techs, from dieticians to physical therapists. You can make each interaction a positive experience or you can "be a pill," as my mother used to say. It helps to realize that although this individual provider is the most important person in *your* life right now, you are only one of dozens of patients who need his or her services. Sometimes you will have to wait—maybe for a long time—because someone with a more urgent need must be treated first. Sometimes your hospital meal might be cold. Your therapist may have just left a child who threw a tantrum. You have the opportunity to decide how you will react. Will you yell or smile? Resolve ahead of time to be as calm and pleasant as you can. Anger interferes with your ability to think and decreases the chances of a helpful response in return.

In our culture of self-esteem, we sometimes yell about everything that is less than perfect. We know how important *we* are, but we may forget how important the other person is. How do you decide when to complain and when to suffer in silence? Probably the worst reason to make a fuss is that you are very upset yourself. Your tolerance for inconveniences will be lower as a result of being ill, and your emotional balance may not be at its best. It is a good idea to give yourself a cooling-off period, if you can, to see if you are still upset the next day. A valid reason for speaking up right away, on the other hand, is to correct anything that has the potential to cause harm to you or to another person. This would include medication errors, unsafe surroundings, or visitors who are ill.

As in the rest of society, there is a chain of command in the health-care setting. It is a matter of respect and fairness to bring your complaint first to the person directly involved in the problem. If you demand to see the hospital administrator before talking to the nurse, you will understandably antagonize her and perhaps damage her reputation unfairly. You only know one side of the story. If, however, your complaint is not taken seriously or falls on deaf ears, you can ask to speak to the supervisor. If that still does not help, speak to your doctor. This is a good time to send "I" messages: I am worried, I want a problem solved, I care about my care. Try to avoid "you" messages: You always bring my meal late, you are too noisy, you are impatient with my questions. These comments have the effect of making the listener defensive and leading you to an argument, not a solution.

Remember, you want to be an effective team member. You can be most effective when you are feeling "put together" and looking your best, whatever that happens to be for that day. Dressing with care and combing your hair can give you additional self-confidence to speak with clarity and assertiveness.

One way you can help yourself is to take care of your surroundings in the hospital so that you feel most comfortable. My physician son calls it "demystifying medical care." You can do a lot to cheer yourself. Consider decorating your hospital room with banners, wall hangings, or an uplifting picture, but don't get in the way of the work areas of the staff. Bring your own clean bathrobe and slippers and maybe a favorite stuffed animal. Ask your doctor if you can bring in snacks that appeal to you—some homemade cookies or muffins, or an ice cream cone delivered by a friend. Music can be soothing, and earphones allow you to choose your music without worry about bothering your roommate. Your own music offers an escape from the daily soap operas. Remember that the health-care setting must be safe for all the patients and staff, so check to be sure your great idea won't be a problem.

In short:

- As a patient you have the right to receive respect and the responsibility to act respectfully when interacting with medical personnel.

- Remember that your provider is helping dozens of patients a day, not just you.

- Think before you complain. Is this a serious health or safety problem or just an annoyance?

- Make your surroundings more "user friendly" with decorations, your own clothing, favorite music with headphones, and familiar food. Check with your doctor first about all of these.

Taming the Red Tape Jungle

In the midst of the initial medical treatments, we'd rather deal with it later than face all of the paperwork and bills. This is an understandable response, but all too soon later arrives and the pile of bills can feel like a ball and chain. Unfortunately the process will remain complex until lawmakers reform the insurance system. In the meantime, you can take some practical steps to keep your sanity in the midst of the deluge of paperwork.

Many of the best programs to help cancer patients with bills require application and acceptance into the program *prior* to the care being delivered. That means it is to your advantage to ask at your oncologist's office or the financial assistance department at your local hospital if they know of any programs that might help with your expenses. Don't wait until you begin receiving big bills and discover that your insurance does not cover the expenses. Being proactive can really help you here.

Most importantly, *keep everything*, even if you just toss it into a cardboard box. Much of the information on the bills is hard to duplicate if the bill has been lost. It will save a lot of time and hassle if you can put your hands on a particular bill from an individual doctor. Happily you almost always have several weeks to several months to figure out what to do about various bills. A system of organizing can really help conserve your energy and sanity.

The key component in my red tape system is a diary. Yours can be as simple or complex as you choose. The essential information is the date, the activity of the day (CT scan, doctor visit, lab tests, surgery) and the providers' names. It is a nuisance to try to remember who did what and when. You need your mind-power for more important things! A simple spiral notebook or a yellow tablet works great. You might want to keep this diary on your cell phone or computer. What makes this system work is to *use it consistently* and *keep it in the same place* so you can find it each time you need it. Leave a few extra blank lines on busier days since you may be billed for services you were not aware of at the time. For example, if you have a surgery, you may receive a bill from the assistant surgeon, the anesthesiologist, the pathologist, the diagnostic laboratory, the hospital, maybe even the emergency room. Make it a habit to write down the day's activities as soon as you get home. This diary is an easy record to refer to several months later. If you don't want to put this together for yourself, you can purchase some of the tracker systems available through bookstores.

Each bill is a separate legal document and must be regarded as a business agreement between you and the provider of care. Once the bills begin to arrive, a filing system can provide at-your-fingertips access to a particular service. I recommend filing bills by provider. (Make note of how you make out the check.) You need a folder or large envelope for each of your doctors, the hospital, the lab, the pharmacy, and the outpatient services you used. You may have additional bills from occupational or physical therapy, counselors, or pathology services. Keep bills in order of date within each folder, with the most recently received in the front.

Do you try to pay your bills as soon as you receive them? In the case of medical care, this may be premature. If you are fortunate enough to be covered partially or fully by insurance, it is often best to wait until your insurance company pays before you send money to the provider. There is usually a delay between the time you receive the bill and the time the insurance company pays their legal share. If you wait until your insurance has paid, the provider will send you another (hopefully smaller) bill, which you can pay then. It simplifies life for everyone and avoids the confusion of refunds and duplicate bills. If you are unsure about what portion of the bill your insurance will cover, you can call either the insurance company or your doctor to ask. This shows that you are a responsible person who intends to pay and that you are doing your best to be conscientious.

What if the amount of the bill is staggering? Sticker shock can be extreme. Health care is frighteningly expensive. Hospitals are struggling just to keep their doors open, so they will charge for everything you use, including oxygen, blood transfusions, aspirin, medications, equipment, and bandaging supplies. It may seem petty to you, but it is a matter of fairness that the person who uses the most in terms of services should pay the cost of that care. Sometimes you may receive a bill for "services rendered" with only one large total charge. (This happens most often with hospitals or similar facilities.) You have the right to request and receive an itemized bill from any care provider. It is emotionally easier to pay the bill when you can see exactly what the costs are and can verify that the bill contains no errors.

If you are a regular customer with your local hospital, it helps a lot to arrange for a personal contact in the billing department. That department may have dozens of employees. It is time-consuming and frustrating to have to explain the same problem, on many occasions, to different people. If you can call and ask for Mrs. Brown (or even better, if you can get her direct line) she will get to know you and much extra explaining will be eliminated. The more she knows your particular case, the easier your life will be. Be as nice as possible and as non-confrontational as you can. Especially with hospital bills the total may be more than you are able to pay immediately. If you have a contact, you may be able to work out an installment payment plan which meets the needs of both parties. This option is seldom offered. You typically will need to *ask* if it is available and sign a contract or agreement that spells out the terms of the payment.

It is even more important to have a personal contact with your insurance company, where hundreds of employees could answer the phones. I was fortunate and delighted to be assigned a caseworker at the insurance company. She was aware of my personal history and my medical needs. She streamlined the pre-authorization process and interceded for me when the insurance denied coverage for care that my doctors considered necessary. It saved me hundreds of dollars, many hours, and a lot of lost sleep to be able to deal with just one person and to have her direct phone line!

What is pre-authorization? Some insurance companies require advance notice of what treatment is planned and why. They must approve care *before* it is given or they will not pay. Insurers vary in their requirements for pre-authorization. Some pay after the treatment, but others require a written request and may take up to two weeks to authorize a procedure before it is given. It is *your* job to know what your insurer requires and to be sure that this pre-approval is received. Check with the person who is scheduling the procedure or call your insurance company yourself. The fine print can be ridiculous. When I was receiving a course of chemotherapy known to extend for eight treatments, three weeks apart, my insurer required a new approval every two months. That meant the doctor's office had to call and be sure that it was OK to continue the treatment plan already in place. My caseworker simplified my life a lot by dealing with these repeated appeals for approval. Fortunately you usually do not need pre-authorization for emergency care.

If your insurance company refuses to pay for services, your doctor's staff can assist you with corrected information or an appeal. Insurance reimbursement is based on at least two complicated numerical systems of codes, one for the disease and one (or more) for the procedures. The same illness can often be described (coded) in multiple ways, and your doctor probably knows which of those true descriptions is most likely to be paid by your particular insurer. If you receive a statement from your insurance company saying a charge was denied, speak first to your provider. Often a staff person who deals all day with insurers can help you get better reimbursement.

Another term you need to know is Explanation of Benefits (EOB). It is a statement from your insurance company letting you know that an insurance claim has been filed, the total amount of the bill, the amount the insurer will pay, the amount that is your share, and the amount that the insurer does not plan to pay, including the reason for the denial. This piece of paper contains a great deal of valuable information. Take these with you to the hospital billing department or your doctor's office any time you need to discuss a bill. Be sure to save them indefinitely!

Plan to deal with money issues when you are thinking the most clearly and feeling your best. For me, that was first thing in the morning on a "good day." This is not a task you want to do on a day when you are suffering from "chemo brain!" I kept a contacts page in each folder with my bills and recorded what happened as I made the calls. Include the day and time, the person you spoke to (name, position, and extension), and your final agreement—I'll call back next Tuesday, the doctor needs to send an additional letter of explanation, etc. Be sure to make a note on your calendar to call back on the agreed-upon date. In general, the longer it takes to resolve questions of payment, the lower your chances of having that decision benefit you. If you appear to be a no-nonsense, businesslike person, you will be taken more seriously. If you have no head for numbers or are easily intimidated, ask a friend to make these calls for you. Expect that you will need to give your permission for him or her to speak on your behalf. This can be as simple as a verbal OK from you while the phone call is in progress. Often you can also request permission for that person to speak for you in future interactions. Ask for an authorization form you can fill out for this purpose, such as an Authorization for Release of Medical Records.

You might find a silver lining to the storm cloud of medical bills. If your bills are high enough in one tax year, you may pay significantly lower federal and state income taxes. The deduction for medical expenses depends on how your medical costs compare to your total income for that year. Keep track of all your expenses from January on each year since a surprise expense may put you into a reduced tax category by December. In addition to the obvious costs of surgery, chemotherapy, and radiation, qualifying medical expenses might include health insurance premiums, eye exams, dental care, transportation for medical treatments, and costs for meals and lodging for distant treatments. Save receipts for every expense and record dates and odometer readings for mileage. Because the IRS system runs on a calendar-year basis, you can consider tax concerns when you are arranging for treatment or paying bills. For instance, if you know your expenses in a given year will be high enough to itemize them, you can schedule routine care such as new glasses or dental work before the end of the calendar year. You may also be able to pay upcoming medical bills before December 31. The IRS considers only when the bill is paid, not when the service was rendered, when figuring the deduction.

Financial red tape is not the only kind you will be dealing with. Your medical history will become more and more complex as you go along, and you will be asked certain questions over and over and over. It really helped my stress level to write down four lists. I still carry them with me at all times.

- List one contains all surgeries and hospital admissions, including the doctor involved, the procedure or illness treated, the date, and the place.

- The second list summarizes all of the medications I take regularly. It lists the exact name copied from the prescription bottle, the dosage, the number of times a day I take the medication, and why I am taking it. It is critical to list any over-the-counter preparations used, including vitamins, calcium tablets, herbal remedies or pain relievers such as aspirin.

- The third list gives the dates of immunizations—tetanus, flu shots, pneumonia vaccine, or anything else.

- The fourth list shows the name and phone number for each of my doctors and for the family member I designate as my emergency contact.

It is stressful to see a new doctor or get emergency care. Having these lists available means you can relax and give the information easily and without worrying about forgetting an important detail. I don't have enough room in my brain to spare for facts that don't need to be carried there!

In short:

- Paperwork will multiply as your treatments progress. A system for dealing with it can save you time, money, and frustration.

- Keep every document related to health care costs.

- A health-care diary is a permanent record of what was done, by whom, on what date.

- File bills and conversations according to provider so you can find the bill you need quickly.

- Wait until your insurance pays their portion before you pay.

- If you cannot afford to pay the bills in full, ask about a payment plan.

- Write down the name, phone number, and extension of your "contact person" at hospitals and insurance companies to avoid having to repeat the same story on each call.

- Deal with money matters when you are most fresh.

- Consider the income-tax implications of your medical care.

- Carry four lists with you at all times:

  - Past surgeries and hospitalizations

  - Dates of immunizations

  - Drugs and non-prescription medications taken

  - Names and phone numbers of your doctors and emergency contacts.

Just Cut It Out!

What if surgery is a part of your treatment plan? Ouch! The very thought brings to mind pain, loss of control, indignities, and unfamiliar places such as hospitals. Naturally no one looks forward to this option; however, in many cases surgery can be curative for cancer, especially if the cancer is localized. In many other cases, surgery is a part of a comprehensive treatment plan that may include chemotherapy or radiation. What can you do to weather the trip if your doctor recommends surgery?

Be informed. Be sure you ask questions, lots of questions, about any part of the experience you worry or wonder about or don't understand. Ask why the surgery is being recommended. Ask exactly what the surgeon expects to do during the surgery. (Realize that this may change during the surgery when he sees what is needed for you.) Will he take out your appendix? Will he remove your colon? Will you have an -ostomy? How will your scar look? Is reconstructive surgery possible or recommended, immediately or later? Will the surgery or reconstruction lead to loss of nerve sensation? Are you a candidate for laparoscopic surgery, which can be easier to tolerate with shorter recovery time? What are your options if you do not have surgery? How much difference will it make? How will you feel when you wake up? What are the risks, in general and in your particular case? Who is the best surgeon to do the surgery you need? What are the long-term limits you may face after your surgery? What kind of anesthesia will be used, and who will administer it? How long will you be in the hospital? How long will you be unable to work or drive? When can the surgery be done?

It is always a good idea to write down your questions in advance of an appointment so that you will not forget an important concern in the fluster of the moment. It is also helpful to bring along a friend or a tape recorder to be sure you hear clearly what the surgeon tells you. (You may be able to use a free cell phone application to do this.) When a person is in a stressful situation—and discussing someone cutting open your body is definitely stressful—it is difficult to think clearly and to organize thoughts well. Take notes.

Now that you are totally overwhelmed by the enormity of the proposed surgery, the most important thing to remember is: Don't panic! Usually your diagnosis is not an emergency, although you certainly want to take action soon. In many cases, your first surgery is the best chance you have to remove all of the cancer, so you want to be well-informed of all the possibilities.

Get a second opinion. Don't worry about hurting the feelings of your original doctors. Many insurance companies *require* a second opinion before they will authorize payment for a surgery. Even if it isn't required, it can be helpful to have the surgery explained by another surgeon. You can be a bit more relaxed about your decision if both surgeons agree. If their recommendations differ, you may want to get a third opinion. Be aware that there are often several different ways to treat a disease, from the most aggressive to the most conservative, and that each approach has benefits and drawbacks. If two doctors recommend different surgeries it does not mean that one is right and the other is wrong. In the final analysis it is *your* body. You will need to decide what treatment is right for you, based on the information you have gathered from your doctors and your research. You will also be the one to live with the results of the surgery, so it is important to take the time you need to be as sure as possible that you have made the best decision for *you*. In most cases a delay of a few days for you to explore options will not have a significant effect on your cancer, and the peace of mind you find may enhance your recovery. Of course, you may need to take action immediately if your cancer surgery is an emergency.

Take good care of yourself while you are waiting for the surgery day, including eating a well-balanced diet. You can add a multivitamin if your diet is less than great. Get as much sleep and exercise as your situation allows. It is also common sense to stay away from anyone who is sick. Your surgery will probably be postponed if you catch a cold or the flu. This is a good time to take advantage of the books and CDs that are available about for preparing for surgery. Some insurance companies offer these for free. Stress relief will make the waiting time easier.

So the big day is tomorrow—what now? Most hospitals have orientation materials that will tell you what to expect and what to bring on the day of your surgery. Many of the rules seem hard-hearted unless you know the reason for them. Usually you will need to report for surgery with an empty stomach, with neither food or liquid in it. As unpleasant as hunger is, the alternative is that you may become nauseated from the surgery and vomit. If you do, the chances of choking or getting pneumonia from inhaling fluid are high and the condition is both life-threatening and miserable. Why won't the hospital let you wear your wedding ring, which you have never removed? Often people experience swelling of the hands during or after surgery. If your hands swell, it may be necessary to cut off that precious ring. Other "spare parts" will need to be removed before your surgery, such as contact lenses, glasses, hearing aids, and removable dental devices of any kind, as well as jewelry including watches or necklaces. It is best to leave them at home or with a family member just for the immediate surgery period. Women will be asked to report with no makeup or nail polish so the anesthesiologist can check your skin color during the surgery and adjust the anesthesia if necessary.

Be prepared for a barrage of repeated questions when you check in for surgery. This duplication is intentional and gives you many opportunities to be sure that *all* of the doctors know *everything* about your medical condition that may play a role in your response to anesthesia or surgery. Something as seemingly insignificant as the aspirin you took for a headache yesterday can have a dramatic effect on your outcome since aspirin can lead to bleeding problems during or after surgery. Be sure to include any herbal or natural food-type supplements. These can also interact with anesthetic agents or other medications. Be as complete as you can in your answers to the questions. Don't let embarrassment keep you from being open and frank in your communication.

After the surgery, you will probably be asked to do some things that you would rather not do—they hurt! Your doctor may ask you to cough. Why in the world would it matter if you cough, when your surgery was done on your abdomen and you feel you will come apart if you cough? One of the most common and deadly complications after surgery is pneumonia. Vigorous coughing will clear the lungs of the mucus that accumulates during surgery and open the airways to allow better exchange of oxygen. You will feel *much* better, much sooner, if you cough. If pain is a serious concern, try pushing a pillow against your incision area when you cough to minimize the motion at that site. Sometimes it helps to draw your knees up to your chest before coughing. You can also do your coughing after you receive pain medication.

Can you believe they are asking you to get up and *walk* right after your surgery? Don't they know you are sick? Walking actually provides many benefits. It is the most effective and safest way known to prevent blood clots in the legs, a serious complication of surgery. It also allows you to maintain whatever physical strength you had going into surgery. Even without surgery, just lying in bed for two or three days results in a wobbly feeling when you do get up. Walking can help keep your fitness level up. Walking can ease the distress of gas pains (which often accompany surgery) by helping your digestive system return to normal sooner. Another benefit is that you will be able to tolerate "real food" sooner. Not so clinical, but also important: Walking gives you a change of scenery and a sense of accomplishment. It is encouraging to see the distance you can walk increase from steps to a few yards, from around the hall once to doing laps. Progress is definite and measurable. When you can control so few things, it is nice to see that you *can* walk. If your surgery does not allow for walking right away, follow the instructions of the staff on what exercises you can do. Again, take pain medicine before you walk, but don't let the pain keep you from walking. You can speed your discharge from the hospital by as much as several days just by doing this. If the nurses seem too busy to help you walk, ask if it is OK for a family member or a friend to accompany you, but *do it*. It is an important part of your recovery.

Another important priority after surgery is to be sure you are eating a well-balanced diet and drinking plenty of fluids. The healing process takes a lot of extra energy (calories) and you will need to fuel your healing by eating well. Your doctor will give you specific dietary instructions, but you will need to commit yourself to eating even if you don't feel like it. Eating is as important as taking prescribed medications! Expect to eat more food and more calories to maintain your weight and to rebuild the tissues disrupted by the surgery. (Don't look at this time of healing as an opportunity for dieting.) Drinking lots of fluids can help protect you against urinary tract infections and constipation, as well as dehydration.

What can you expect as you recover at home? You should be prepared for some pain, which should get progressively better. You will have some tenderness at the site of the surgery for several months as your body mends. Eventually you will have a painless scar, although that can seem far away in the days right after the surgery.

You may have some minor bleeding and maybe some drainage of fluids, especially if you have a drain placed during surgery. A drain is simply a plastic tube, usually sutured to your skin, which leads the fluid out from the surgery area to a bulb or bandage. The drain allows fluid buildup to escape rather than accumulating under your skin. If the fluid is not drained, it can lead to infection or additional tissue damage. Drains are almost always used on a temporary basis. Swelling and redness are variable, depending on the type of surgery you have. They may be minimal or significant, short-lived or slow to resolve.

For all of these situations—pain, redness, swelling, and drainage or bleeding—the important questions to ask are these: "Is this symptom better than it was yesterday or an hour ago? Is it the same? Or are any of these symptoms worse now than they were before?" A change for the worse means you need to call your surgeon to determine if you are developing an infection or if you have a problem with wound healing. You may need a change in pain medication or an antibiotic.

Some of the aftereffects of surgery are not localized to the wounded area. Your whole body had an assault on its resources, and you can expect to feel wiped out. It takes a great deal of energy for your body to heal those damaged cells and tissues, to clear away cellular debris, to keep your immune system alert to infections, and to regain flexibility and normal use. You should expect fatigue to be part of your recovery—it is your body's way of telling you to slow down and let the healing take place. This is a great time to listen to your body. When you are tired, *rest!* Rest may mean a few minutes on the couch or a two-hour nap, but you will get better faster and with less pain if you are aware of your physical needs and respect them.

Along the same lines, you can expect to have some emotional unevenness. Some patients, particularly the frail or those having extensive surgery, may experience a phenomenon known as "sundowning." This condition is seen most often at the end of the day or during the night. The patient sees things that are not there, hears voices, or becomes paranoid. No one knows the exact cause of the syndrome, but most often it resolves on its own as recovery progresses. If it happens to you, be assured that you are not crazy, just recovering from surgery!

Maybe you are usually a stoic person; suddenly you break into tears for no reason at all. Perhaps you are usually "on top of things" and organized; now you feel disoriented and distracted, and find it hard to concentrate. You may feel euphoric for a time—hugely relieved that the surgery is successfully behind you—only to find yourself plunged into despondency the same afternoon. It's OK! This is normal! It is normal for all surgery patients, even those having cosmetic or elective surgery. It is particularly hard to avoid if your surgery was done to treat or remove a cancer. You will have all the systemic ups and downs of hormone levels, pain relievers, and blood-sugar level fluctuations. You are also dealing with the vivid awareness that your cancer diagnosis is real, and cancer is having a disturbing and immediate effect on your life. It's hard to pretend that everything is OK when you are recovering from surgery, even though it may well be that your surgery has removed all of the cancer.

One last word about fatigue and emotional responses. Often you will be so excited when you begin to feel better that you enthusiastically tackle too much. It is so tempting to overdo! And you may not realize that you have done too much until you suddenly collapse, either with exhaustion or in tears. This is a learning experience! Take it more slowly next time. If you have great self-control, you may be able to avoid this downswing by gradually increasing your activity by no more than ten to twenty-five percent a day. It really is more fun to see yourself steadily improving than to do too much and regret it.

In short:

- Be informed. Ask all of the questions that occur to you

and write down both questions and answers.

- Get a second opinion, if appropriate. Surgery is often irreversible, and it pays to think first.

- Before surgery, keep healthy by eating well, sleeping enough, and exercising. Avoid sick friends.

- Follow the rules, especially about food and liquid limitations before surgery and removing jewelry, dentures, and contact lenses.

- Be honest and complete. Tell your doctors everything! Better to be embarrassed than to have a bad reaction because of a medication or herb you didn't mention.

- After surgery, follow directions exactly in terms of exercise, walking, or coughing.

- Eat well to provide fuel for the healing process.

- Call your surgeon if pain, redness, swelling, drainage, or bleeding is greater than expected.

- Be prepared to be very tired as you recover, and take time to rest.

- Emotional instability is often a sign that you are doing too much.

Missing Pieces?

For some of the most common cancers, surgery can result in losing a part of your body. Patients treated for cancer of the breast, prostate, colon, bladder, testes and ovaries, or those who lose a limb, are particularly vulnerable to changes in self-image and self-confidence as a result of their treatment. Somehow, loss of a part of your lung or muscle seems less threatening to who you are than loss of a limb, a nose, a breast, or a sexual organ. Loss of normal bodily functions (sexual responses, bladder control, or bowel control) requires a big adjustment. You can deal with "just an operation" if you look the same and feel the same, although more sore! What if your body *doesn't* look or behave the way it did before treatment? (If you are not in this situation, you may prefer to skip this chapter.)

First of all, it helps to remember that your identity is an interior thing. Your unique self is the sum of your genetic background, your culture, your education, your family upbringing, and your own experiences. Your body is the vehicle, but *you* are the engine that makes the whole thing run. Even if the vehicle changes, you have the capacity to continue through life in a way that has meaning for you and those around you. You just drive around in a more distinctive chassis!

Even if you are the same inside, you may experience profound grief if you lose a body part. Some people feel devastated. In fact, this fear of losing a part can lead patients to refuse treatment. They may say, "I would rather die than live without—a leg, a breast, my sexual function." Almost always the choice to preserve a cancerous part leads to death from the cancer sooner than if it is treated or surgically removed. Still, it is *your* body, and you do have the right to make this choice. That's why your surgery permit always includes a full explanation of the planned surgery. Your signature shows that you understand and agree to the procedure *and* the resulting limitations.

What if you did understand and agree to the surgery but afterward you are overwhelmed with the enormity of what was done? There is no going back. Cosmetic surgery can help with appearance but some decisions are irreversible, such as losing ovaries, testes, or your colon. The implications are huge for you and your spouse, for today and the future.

Let's start with you, today. After any surgery, you will be provided with a way to cope with the changes. You may have an "-ostomy," an artificial opening in the skin that collects urine or feces in a small, easily concealed, disposable bag. You may be fitted with a prosthesis, an artificial limb or breast. You may need to use a walker or a wheelchair, short or long term. You will be dealing with major changes in your personal habits in every case. Especially at first, when you are still recovering physically and emotionally from the trauma of surgery itself, these new challenges can feel insurmountable. You may feel clumsy, ugly, or even repulsive. This is the time to talk to a survivor! It is so important to meet someone who has come through the challenge and now is poised, confident, and happy again. He or she can reassure you that everyone suffers at least some level of depression over the changes, but that time and healing can restore you to sanity. Your doctors can give you a professional opinion, but nothing compares to the reassurance of seeing someone who has "been there." If you don't know anyone, ask your doctor for the name of a person with an experience similar to yours.

Our sense of masculinity or femininity can take a beating, too. If you are already feeling down, you may find yourself taking less care with your appearance, which tends to make you feel even worse. It's easy to slip into a pattern of skimping on your usual grooming routines by not shaving or washing your hair. The opposite approach, paying even more attention to your appearance, is much more helpful. It gives you a lift every time you look in the mirror and reassures your family and friends that you are still you. Many cancer patients are reluctant to purchase new, attractive clothing for themselves because they are worried about "wasting" the money or the clothing if they do not live long enough to wear out the item. Many of your current clothes can still suit you, but purchasing one or two new things can give your sense of sexuality a much-needed boost.

What about your spouse? He or she will need to make a major adjustment to the new you. The most supportive spouse in the world still notices and cares about the ways you are different. It is human nature to resist change. Fortunately it is also human nature to adapt, to be flexible, to grow. Conflict can arise if the patient adapts more or less quickly than the spouse. It is painful for both partners when the patient is ready to move on to new ways of expressing intimacy but the spouse is still deeply grieving, or vice versa. This is a transforming time in a relationship. Over a period of weeks or months, you will redefine yourself, your partner, your own sexuality, and your spouse's sexuality. It is a long-term process. Actually it is a lifelong process. Great patience is required, since each person can only move forward and change at the pace that is right for him or her. Perhaps the only thing that can help is to experiment, to be adventurous, to be willing to find out what works and also what doesn't work. This is a good time to try new things. Give honest feedback to each other. Our sexuality can be expressed and enhanced in so many ways. Some variables to consider: clothing, makeup, lighting, scents, music, foods, jewelry, touch, massage, or a change of scene. Remember, the most important sexual organ is the brain!

One issue that may come up during your treatment is your future ability to have children. Removal of ovaries or testes results in infertility. Sometimes chemotherapy or radiation can result in either short-term infertility or permanent sterility. Surgery or radiation for prostate cancer can result in impotence. Check with your doctor about your options if you are hoping to have children in the future. Many organizations can help you with information, including Fertile Hope. Discuss the possibilities with your mate as soon as you realize it will be an issue and get counseling if you face conflicts here. Our ability to have children is often close to the heart of our life's dreams. The grieving can be intense, and you may need help to sort it all out.

In short

- Losing a body part is intensely emotional. It can affect your sense of self and of sexuality.

- You may experience profound grief and may benefit from professional help to sort this out.

- Many devices can enable patients with -ostomies or missing body parts to continue to lead normal, active, productive lives. Talk with a survivor!

- Your spouse will also be dealing with redefining the relationship—be patient with both of you!

- Discuss fertility issues as soon as you realize they are a concern.

- Be flexible. Experiment. Laugh.

- Extra efforts to look your best definitely pay off in a happier spirit.

- Remember that you are much more than the body you use.

Chemotherapy, Up Close and Personal

❧❧❧

Chemotherapy, often shortened to chemo, is one of the most terrifying words in the English language. We have an unfortunate tendency to completely overlook the "therapy" part of the word and to feel powerless in the face of impersonal chemistry. It doesn't help that many of us have known someone treated with chemotherapy, often many years ago, who became very ill from the treatments. If chemo is part of the journey you face, how do you cope?

The first priority here, as with all components of your healing regimen, is to deal with your fear. By now you are getting good at that! Recognize that the shaking knees, inability to concentrate, and sense of disconnectedness you may experience during the initial discussion with your oncologist are symptoms not of your cancer, but of your preconceived ideas about this "chemo monster." Remember that before your diagnosis your cancer was just as real, you simply were unaware of the problem. Now that you *are* aware, you are empowered to act.

How can you begin to tame this fear? It helps if you can determine the source. What experiences or stories from your life, even as a child, are contributing to your fear? I realized that both my mother and father died of cancer and both received chemotherapy. In my mind, chemotherapy equaled death. I was unaware of the huge advances in the last several decades. When I recognized the thought process, I was able to ask my oncologist directly, "What are the chances that this treatment will kill me?" His honest answer, "Very unlikely!" gave me the inner confidence to say, "The potential benefits for me outweigh the potential risk." *He* already knew that but *I* needed to accept those risks for myself, as a conscious decision. Maybe you fear losing your hair (you may or may not, see Chapter 15, Hair Today, Gone Tomorrow) or feeling sick or losing your job or being unable to care for yourself or others. Each of us knows, deep inside, what our primary fear is. If we name it (i.e., the fear of losing my job), look at it in the light of day (might this really happen?) and imagine the consequences (OK, so I might be unemployed), then we can ask, could I survive this? Would I be "OK," even in this worst-case scenario? Most often we know we *could* be OK, even though the outcome would not be our choice. Accepting the fears and the risks can lead to a peaceful heart during treatment, a wonderful boost to our overall health.

It is important to carefully choose your medical oncologist (the doctor who specializes in chemotherapy and other interventional medical treatments). He or she will be your tour guide on this wild ride. A vast amount of data is available and it is constantly being updated. You want an oncologist who is well-informed, willing to collaborate with colleagues to plan your course of treatment, and able to explain clearly and compassionately to you what lies ahead. I felt like I had a tiger by the tail! It took every bit of my attention, energy, focus, and cooperation, along with every bit of my doctor's expertise, to receive the optimum benefit from my treatments. A sense of collaboration and teamwork between the doctor and patient is crucial here. This is not the time for a doctor who pats your head and says, "There, there. Everything will be OK. Just trust me." It is equally unhelpful to have a doctor who tells you in exquisite detail about every possible complication you may encounter. I found the best balance to be a physician who is knowledgeable, honest, and encouraging but who responds to patient questions rather than giving a canned speech. This allows the patient to control the rate at which information is taken in, based on his or her intellectual, emotional, and physical state at that moment. Some days I preferred no additional data at all since I was already overloaded. Other days I felt prepared to deal with those nagging worries by asking the questions. It takes a lot of courage to ask. It is easier to say, "Just do it," but I am convinced that the full consent of the patient is a key factor in how well the treatment goes. By "consent" I don't mean legal permission. Your consent must result from weighing the options and freely choosing chemotherapy based on your conviction that it is in your overall best interest. This consent takes into account all the variables of your life, including physical needs, emotional health, family, job, and lifestyle.

As you are choosing your oncologist, be sure to ask if he or she is willing for you to bring a caregiver or a friend to your appointments who can either tape-record or take notes of the conversation so you can check back later on exactly what was said.

Your physician is required by law to inform you in broad terms what to expect. A good oncologist, however, will emphasize that every chemotherapeutic agent is unique, every cancer is unique, and every body responds in its own way to the treatments. Chemotherapy is not a description of a universal medicine in the sense that aspirin is a treatment for all inflammation. Chemotherapy refers to any one or combination of *dozens* of drugs acting in a variety of ways to block, slow, or kill cancerous cells. The chemo agents chosen for you and their dosage, strength, interval between treatments, and route of administration (oral, intravenous, or intraperitoneal) will be specific for your needs, based on a whole variety of factors. These include your overall health, body size, age, and ongoing treatments for other problems such as high blood pressure, diabetes, and allergies. Each treatment plan is specific for your *particular* tumor and takes into account the type of tumor (sarcoma, carcinoma, etc.), the site of the tumor (colon, breast, prostate), the stage of the tumor (is it localized or has it spread to nearby or distant organs), and most importantly, what agents are most effective for your kind of cancer. It's an amazing puzzle your oncologist must research on your behalf! The treatment plan that results should be the best possible fit for you. In larger hospitals, your case may be presented to a "tumor board," a group of doctors that includes pathologists, surgeons, radiation oncologists, and medical oncologists, who will discuss the specific recommendations each believes to be best for your individual case.

An awareness of the complexity involved in setting up a chemotherapy regimen helped me avoid the temptation to compare my treatment plan or progress with anyone else. It is important to recognize that some "self-help" sources of information, such as books and especially the Internet, offer advice that does not take into account all of the important variables for your particular case. If you want to do your own research, I urge you to check the credentials of every source of information and to *ask your own doctor* about any treatment you believe may hold promise for you. This will not only protect you from financial burdens you don't need but can also warn you of possible harmful interactions with your ongoing treatments. Chemotherapy can suppress your normal immune system responses. Avoid putting yourself at additional risk by taking unknown preparations.

Be prepared to hear the response "We don't know" a lot. Will this treatment cure me? We don't know. Will I suffer from (nausea, headache, tingling feet, etc.)? We don't know. Will I be able to keep working during treatments? Will I catch more colds? We don't know. It is possible to say *some* people respond in a certain way, but you are unique!

Perhaps more than any other kind of medical care, chemotherapy treatments are based on a feedback cycle.

The oncologist develops an overall plan, but your physical (and in some cases, emotional) response to the treatments determines whether, and how, that schedule will be modified. Maybe a side effect becomes more worrisome than the cancer—the agent may be changed. Maybe your tumor, measured by various tests, is responding better or more quickly than expected. Maybe a research study just published shows that eight treatments are as effective as twelve. (This actually happened to me—I was ecstatic!) Maybe your blood counts are too low for a scheduled treatment and you are given a week off. Sometimes your reactions are caused by pre-medications, not the chemotherapy itself. For instance, steroids can lead to hyperactivity or sleep disruptions, and Benadryl can cause blurry vision or spacey thinking. In these cases, too, adjustments can often be made.

The key point is that you, the patient, are the only one who can report accurately the information needed to adjust your treatments. I am forever grateful to my oncologist for his comment right at the beginning that there is no correlation between the severity of side effects and the effectiveness of the treatment. Since that is so, it clearly makes sense to minimize the side effects. Don't be shy! Don't worry that you will be considered a whiner. Don't let fear stop you! Be honest, as accurate as possible (is this a minor inconvenience or a major disruption?) and as quantitative as possible (Do I feel this way once in a while? All the time? Is it getting worse? Only on day three?). I learned as I went along that many side effects can be helped or eliminated if your doctor knows about them. If you just suffer in silence, you may very well be suffering unnecessarily. As I went through my chemo times, I saw myself as a partner with my doctor, working toward the common goal of my healing. His job was to know the options and keep me as comfortable as possible while treating me for maximum effect. *My* job was to report anything that caught my attention along the way. At first I tried to decide for myself what changes were or were not important. Eventually I learned to make notes about everything. My doctor knew that if it was a problem of no significance or something unavoidable, I would be satisfied with that answer. Sometimes the problems I thought I just had to endure (for instance, nausea or tingling feet) could actually be treated quite effectively. Ask!

You may be at increased risk for infection because chemotherapy can interfere with your immune system by depleting white blood cells. A simple cold is no big deal when you are otherwise well, but if you are immune-suppressed it can quickly lead to pneumonia. It is important for you to be aware of your exposure to disease organisms. Avoid people who are obviously sick or situations where many people are packed together. Washing your hands many times a day is one of the best things you can do to stay well. Call your oncologist at the *first* sign of an infection! Immediate treatment is often needed to prevent the infection from becoming much worse in a matter of hours. Signs of infection are fever (over 100.5 degrees), sore throat, cough, redness, open sores, swelling, vomiting, or diarrhea. If you think you might have an infection, *call right away*, even during non-office hours, even if your own oncologist is gone. A doctor is always on call. Be sure you explain that you are getting chemotherapy and you might have an infection. This is a problem that will not wait. If you are instructed to go to the emergency room, *go*. You aren't being brave to avoid this trip; you are being foolish.

The day of your chemotherapy treatment, you can do several things to make yourself more comfortable. Drinking lots of water before you arrive makes it much easier to start an IV line. It also gives you a head start on the advice you usually receive, "Drink lots of water." Experience will show you what kind of meal to eat before a treatment. In general, a light meal of non-fatty, non-acidic food is best. Treatment may take several hours. Bring along something to help pass the time—a friend to chat with, a craft project, a good book, music on CD or a DVD (with player and headphones). I found that collections of short stories were best for me, since I sometimes had fuzzy vision or fuzzy thinking. Some patients have a "port" implanted under their skin for ease of access for the chemotherapy. If you have a port, you may find that using an ice pack during the car ride to the treatment center will numb the skin just enough to make the needle stick a lot easier. If the access site varies for you, ask about the numbing sprays that are available. Comfortable, non-binding clothes are a good idea. If you have a port, be sure your clothing will allow access and avoid pullover shirts. You might want to bring along a snack, lunch, or a can of your favorite soda. Your treatments may result in feelings of chill or warmth so dress in layers and ask for a warm blanket if you need one.

Many books have been written about dealing with the side effects of chemotherapy. If you are having any problem, first ask your oncologist for recommendations about things you can do to ease the situation. Then give his or her suggestions a fair try. Many times a long-term benefit is achieved by choosing to do something unpleasant in the short term. For example, I found that nausea was greatly reduced for me if I constantly sipped water or cider during the hours right after chemo, although right then drinking did not appeal to me at all. In cases like this, being good to your body means choosing the action you know is best for you, regardless of how you feel about doing it. I believe each of us has an inner "knowing," an awareness of what is in our body's best interest. Too often, we make ourselves sick by ignoring that inner voice or intuition—by eating too much, working too much, or sitting too much—and we suffer as a result.

If possible, plan treats for yourself to take advantage of the days when you feel great and to give yourself something to look forward to. I would make a date to have lunch with a friend, go to a play, or take a long drive. You can always cancel if you don't feel up to it when the time comes. Making no plans because you might feel sick is a bleak way to live. Look ahead to fun!

In short:

- Get all of the information you want/need about your chemotherapy agents.

- Your treatment plan is specifically formulated for you. You cannot compare your course with that of anyone else.

- Your oncologist requires your feedback to provide the best care. Be honest and complete when you report side effects or difficulties.

- The day of chemo, pay special attention to food, water, diversion, and clothing choices.

- Avoid sick people and immediately report any signs of an infection to your doctor.

- Plan a reward for each treatment cycle.

Hair Today, Gone Tomorrow?

❧❧❧

Some people really aren't affected by their hair—there or gone, it's all the same to them. If you have this attitude, read no further.

If you are like the vast majority of us, when you look in the mirror you expect to see someone familiar looking back. A significant part of our self-image is the location, color, and style of our hair. It can be a great jolt to find some or all of it missing, even temporarily. Even though we are forewarned, even though we consciously chose to have the potentially life-saving treatment that resulted in the hair loss, it is still a shock. The shock has several components. How do I look to myself? How do I look to others? How does this affect my identity?

First, let's deal with self-image. From the time we can remember, we are accustomed to including our hair as part of who we are. We describe ourselves on our driver's licenses as having red, blond, or brown hair. We carefully consider haircuts, styles, and color and many of us, especially women, spend a lot of money and time to arrange our hair in a way that flatters our face and figure. We agonize over a bad haircut, one that makes us look "funny," and can't wait for it to grow out. It is almost beyond our imagination how we would look without hair. We are attached to our facial hair, too, and part of our expressiveness comes with our use of a raised eyebrow or a mustache to stroke. Looking in the mirror and seeing no fuzz at all can be very disconcerting.

Secondly, the way others perceive us is important to most people. Men may consider their new look distinguished. Women, who rarely have to deal with balding in the normal course of events, may see a bald head as a beacon shouting, "Cancer! Cancer!" People may be looking at us with pity in their eyes at the exact time that we would prefer to go about our business in as normal a way as possible. They may open the door for us, carry our sweater, or pick up the "doggie bag" at the restaurant, as if we have suddenly become incompetent. In addition to the immediate effect of our baldness on our family and our friends, we may fear that even after our hair grows back our friends will have an indelible mental picture of us at our least attractive.

What are the options? Some people actually feel so strongly about the indignity of hair loss that they refuse treatment on that basis, opting either for no treatment or for an agent that does not have this side effect. Fortunately other alternatives can help to get through the hair loss with reasonable sanity and appearance. Your radiation oncologist or medical oncologist will probably warn you before the start of treatment if hair loss is possible or probable for you. If he or she doesn't mention this at the time of the initial discussion, *ask*. This is not the sort of surprise you need, and much can be done to soften the impact by planning ahead.

If you are aware that hair loss may occur for you, you have several alternatives.

Some patients go to a wig or beauty supply store as soon as they know there may be a need, to begin the process of selecting a wig to use for a period of several weeks or months. It's a lot more fun (you may even find yourself laughing out loud!) if you take your spouse, a daughter, or a good buddy. The advantage of going in early is that the stylist can help you choose a wig that is most similar to your natural hair in color, style, and texture. Some wigs may need to be ordered, and if you plan ahead, the wig can arrive before you need it. A wig can look so real that even those who know you will be unaware that you are wearing it. I'll never forget a male friend's comment to me, "You look terrific! What's different? It must be your hair." I didn't have the heart to tell him it was a wig. Wigs can be sized, cut and styled to your preferences. Obviously a mistake won't grow back, so be sure to go to a stylist who is familiar with working on wigs!

In general, wigs are fairly easy to care for, but there are a few things I wish I had known. If yours is made from a synthetic fiber, be very careful with heat. The blast of hot air from opening an oven or barbeque can frizz your locks with no chance for repair Also be aware of special hairsprays formulated for use on wigs, and don't just use the leftover hair spray on your bathroom shelf. An inexpensive wig stand can protect your style between uses or overnight. Some beauty supply stores give a discount on wigs to people who are losing their hair due to cancer treatments—be sure to ask. Some insurance covers the cost if your doctor writes a prescription. Again, just ask. Your local chapter of the American Cancer Society or your infusion center often have free used wigs available.

Another option is to simply "go natural" and live with a bald head for however long is necessary. Several friends chose to wear a pink ribbon, the kind made for baby girls, around their bald head and simply incorporated their new look into their wardrobe. Maybe you are more comfortable using the scarf solution. Several excellent videos, DVDs, and YouTube videos show a variety of creative ways to make your head covering part of a stunning outfit. Another alternative is to add flair to your usual clothing choices with a collection of hats in various colors, styles, and fabrics. The American Cancer Society publishes a catalog called *TLC* that offers many practical, flattering and reasonably priced hats and scarves. (Call your local American Cancer Society to get on their mailing list.) Many women use a combination of approaches, depending on the day, the weather, and their mood.

How do you get from hair to there? You can let nature take its course and watch as the hair gradually thins or falls out over a period of a few days This approach has the advantage that if some of your hair remains attached, you can make the most of it. Some patients prefer a proactive approach and either get a very short haircut or shave their head in advance of the loss. Few decisions regarding your cancer journey are as personal and emotional as this one. Take the time to listen to your heart to decide just what *you* choose to do. Do not be swayed by family members or doctors! This can be a difficult adjustment, and you will feel better about it if *you* have taken control of how you will respond.

You may have some scalp tenderness (it feels a bit like a sunburn) during the time of hair loss, but it usually is better in a few days. Once your hair is gone, a variety of practical tips can make the time more pleasant. I was surprised to learn how chilly my head would be without hair. You may want to wear a soft, ski-type hat to bed or when outdoors just to retain body heat in the winter. In summer, the opposite problem of overheating can be minimized by wearing lightweight cotton bandana-type scarves that protect you from sunburn and yet still breathe. Enjoy the freedom of swimming without hair in your eyes!

Be very careful about the sun. You will need to consistently use sunscreen. Remember to apply it to the area where your eyebrows used to be, as well as to the rest of your face. I had a scorcher of an eyebrow sunburn one spring! Not only will the sunscreen protect you from the damaging rays, but it will also minimize the tan line that tends to form at the edge of a hat or scarf. If you want just a *little* color for your face and head, consider very short, very *careful*, late day or early morning exposures of both your face and head to the sun. If you can avoid a tan line, you will be able to discard the head coverings sooner when your hair begins to grow back in.

Some treatments cause the loss of eyebrows and eyelashes. If yours does, you can encourage those hairs to stay in as long as possible by treating them gently, not washing them vigorously or using an abrasive or hard eyebrow pencil. A number of professional beauty products can help camouflage these areas once lashes and brows have fallen out. I recommend the "Look Good, Feel Better" programs presented free to cancer patients by the American Cancer Society. These programs offer expert advice on applying makeup to cancer-sensitive skin and top-quality cosmetic products at no charge.

When your hair begins to grow back, it may be different from the way you remember it. Besides being a whole lot shorter, it may be curlier, coarser, thicker, thinner, or a different color. If your new hair is grayer than you prefer, it can be fun to experiment with semi-permanent hair dyes now. Darker colors tend to show up more and you will feel you have more hair if you can see it. If it grows in curly, this may or may not be permanent. Often the curls will last only for the first couple of inches, then the hair will revert to straight if that is your natural tendency. The challenge is to find a hairstyle that suits you for each stage of the growing-out process. A good hair stylist can trim just the edges and around the ears and give even a half-inch worth of hair a look of style and neatness. (My husband called my new hairdo "chic"!) It can be difficult to let scissors touch that precious new hair, but the sense of assurance and style that results is worth the loss of a bit of hair.

How did I handle the challenge of hair loss? The first time around, I was most concerned with my daughter's reaction since she was a typical thirteen-year-old who spent long hours taking care of her own hair. I knew that seeing me bald would intensify the impact of my illness on her. So I took her with me to shop for a wig (before hair loss) and we laughed together at the prospect of me as a redhead! I chose a wig in a color and style that looked as much as possible like my own hair. I wore the wig consistently for many months, since I hoped people would forget that it was a wig if I didn't alternate between a wig and hats or scarves. It eased my sense of being different and conspicuous. No one except my husband saw me without my wig. After my second chemo, I was much less concerned with what other people thought and much more at ease knowing that the hair really would grow back. I alternated between scarves, hats, and the wig, depending on my physical and emotional comfort that particular day. By that time, two years later, I had also discovered that being different was not such a bad thing and that my distinctive appearance opened doors of conversation and allowed me to encourage others. What helped me most was my belief that a big smile would be more memorable to the people around me than my missing hair, so I smiled all the time!

If your hair loss is total, you may lose underarm, pubic, chest, and leg hairs as well as facial and scalp hair. Again, this challenge can impact self-image. It helps to remember that this is a temporary situation. You are the same wonderful person on the inside, where it counts most.

In short:

- Losing your hair can be one of he most emotionally challenging parts of cancer treatment.

- You can decrease the impact by choosing for yourself how you plan to deal with it: a short buzz cut in advance, a wig, hats, scarves, or a bow.

- Protect your eyebrows and lashes before loss by using makeup gently or not at all.

- Be especially careful to use sunscreen!

- Your hair may grow back thicker, thinner, grayer, curlier, or a different color from before. These changes can be temporary or permanent.

- A big smile lifts your spirits and will make a greater impact than your missing hair.

Radiation Therapy Survival Tips

❧❧❧

Radiation therapy uses beams of X-rays to damage and kill cancer cells. It may be used alone or in combination with chemotherapy drugs or surgery. It can be used to completely eradicate a cancer or to slow or control tumor growth or symptoms.

If your cancer is highly susceptible to the effects of radiation or is quite small, the radiation may be the only treatment you receive and may result in a cure. More often, radiation is used in combination with surgery or with chemotherapy to minimize the size of the tumor. For breast cancer and prostate cancer, the two most common cancers treated with radiation, the course of therapy (the total cumulative dose of radiation) is usually determined at the beginning, and the treatments are spread out over a period of several weeks of short daily treatments. You may hear a patient say, "I have twenty-eight treatments to go" based on this kind of advance planning. Newer treatment regimens may allow a higher dose to be delivered for fewer days to certain patients who qualify for the therapy, depending on their tumor type, stage, and location. The treatment schedule may be altered because every person's response to the radiation is different. Sometimes a rest period is advised to allow side effects to ease before the treatments resume. The aim is still the same, to administer the optimum cumulative dose.

Your reaction to radiation treatments will be determined by your past experiences and your unique personality. Many patients zip right through it. Because I found it a challenge, I want to share the tips that helped me.

The concept is beguilingly simple. The patient just needs to lie there, hold still, and allow the radiation beam to focus on the area of cancer to kill the offending cells with as little damage as possible to the healthy surrounding tissue. Maybe because it sounds so easy, the intensity of my emotional response to radiation treatments caught me by surprise. I found myself on the treatment table, motionless and weeping. Why was I so upset? It took me several months of reflection after treatment ended to recognize the causes of my distress.

In a physical sense, it certainly was easy to present myself for treatments. What is difficult is the emotional challenge of the losses that are involved: loss of control, loss of tactile comfort, loss of privacy, and loss of pretense. Each of these may be disturbing, and each patient may experience them to some degree.

Loss of control refers to the ability of the patient to participate in his or her own therapy and therapy decisions. Most of us have some familiarity with the concept of medications and can understand the wisdom of surgery. On the other hand, few people are familiar with the concepts of radiation, the units of dosage, and the mathematics involved in determining fields of treatment. From the beginning, therefore, the patient must choose to place blind trust in the competence of the radiation oncologist who is directing the treatment. You simply must have faith that he or she has the knowledge and ability to provide the care that is best for you. Even after treatments are in progress, the patient cannot do much to reassure himself that all is going well. When you are getting a chemo drug you can look at the IV bottle to be sure the name of the drug and the dosage amount are correct. As you listen to the whirring of the machine, however, you can only hope that the dials and numbers were properly set. You have nothing to see or verify, no scar to examine, no tangible indication that all is well. The built-in distance of this mode of therapy is especially uncomfortable if a patient has grown more and more accustomed to participating in his or her own treatment.

The loss of tactile comfort sounds like a childish thing to notice, but there it is: It is just not as pleasant to lie down on a cold, hard table as it is to sit in a soft recliner or be tucked into a freshly made hospital bed. Your whole body is aware that this is the opposite of "warm and fuzzy." In our daily routines we are used to a padded existence as couch potatoes, not to sitting or lying on a hard, cold table. In addition to the hardness of the surface, the body may need to be positioned with a variety of molds or braces to allow the radiation beams to pass exactly where they should. Perhaps an arm may be up over your head, held in place by a wooden or plastic support. Added to the cold, hard machinery feel may be the loss of human touch, something we associate, consciously or unconsciously, with health care. In almost every other healing setting, the patient is touched: a pulse is felt, an IV is started, a stethoscope is placed, a hand supports you. In this setting, you may be well enough to climb up on the table by yourself, to position yourself, and to climb down unassisted. You can leave each day without ever touching another human being. It is as if you, a human, have intruded into the realm of machines and the machines make all the rules. Fortunately this loss of tactile comfort can be offset by your comfort choices, as I'll discuss below.

The third kind of loss that can add to the emotional challenge of radiation treatment is loss of privacy. Many patients come in and out and are treated for relatively short intervals. This rapid turnover may tempt technicians to act with efficiency rather than with concern for your modesty. If you are lying on a cold, hard, table in the middle of a cold room with your arm over your head and your breast exposed when a strange man walks in to get some clean sheets out of the cabinet, you may feel trapped. There is nowhere to go: You cannot move or you will change the position of the treatment field, and you can't even grab for a blanket. Sometimes the best you can do is to pretend that either you or the unknown person isn't really there, that this isn't happening. Your emotions may object to this intrusion even if your rational mind is telling you that you are receiving medical treatment and there is no need to be embarrassed. In most cases, medical care that requires the patient to be undressed is provided in a setting that is somewhat controlled. In a hospital room, for instance, a drape is drawn closed; in an office, the exam room door is closed. The people present are usually just the doctor or nurse, and the space around the patient is relatively small. The radiation oncology department, however, requires large rooms to accommodate bulky machines, and space constraints sometimes result in the rooms being "multi-purpose." Knowing the staff members are used to seeing many patients a day in various stages of exposure brought me little comfort. It can seem that all of the people who walk in are observers of your private experience. Again, this concern will be addressed below.

Maybe the most difficult of all of the losses, however, is the last: Loss of pretense. The pretense lost here is the myth, "I'm really OK, and I look OK, so no one will know I have cancer." For example, many breast cancer patients wear a prosthesis or have had reconstruction, cover their scars, dress with style, and look normal to everyone around them. It is easy to pretend that because you *look* fine, you *are* fine. On the treatment table, however, with nothing but your skin to shield your brokenness, it is impossible to pretend that things are normal. Simply showing up to Radiation Oncology is a daily reminder that you are not well, you *do* have a serious health problem, and you do *not* know the ultimate resolution of your cancer. If your chemotherapy treatments are on a twenty-one-day cycle, you can forget for two and a half weeks or so that you are locked in a battle with cancer. Your daily radiation appointment is a constant, unremitting reminder that you are mortal—and wounded, at that.

You can begin to take charge of your emotional comfort on your first visit with your radiation oncologist. Ask to see the treatment rooms. Knowing what to expect and having time to adjust to the idea definitely helps. Be sure to ask questions and ask to see the calculations or the diagrams that are part of your treatment plan. Even if you don't understand—and you probably won't!—it is reassuring to actually set eyes on the work that has been done on your behalf.

In general, your first exposure to the equipment (no pun intended) is a simulation, which involves taking several X-rays to localize the tumor area and establish the proper machine settings. This can take an hour or two. Markings on your skin are necessary for the accurate alignment of the machines. You may have this done with markers, which must be very carefully protected from washing off, or with tattoos, which are tiny but permanent dots. During the simulation, it is good to ask if it is possible in your particular case to shield sensitive areas. Your doctor may be able to shield areas near the tumor site, such as the esophagus or axilla in the case of breast cancer, to minimize side effects in those areas.

Once treatment starts, you will usually see a technician for daily treatments. Most treatment sessions only take fifteen minutes or so, although this will depend on your particular cancer. (You can expect that the length of time for each treatment will be fairly consistent, however.) Ask questions if anything is out of the usual routine. This is, after all, your health at stake. It is much better to ask ten times and be assured that nothing is wrong than to not ask once and miss a problem. Speak up if something is upsetting you or if your body is in an uncomfortable position. Often a minor adjustment can make a major difference in your comfort.

You will probably see your radiation oncologist about once a week or more often if you have questions or a problem arises. This appointment will take longer than your treatment alone since it usually involves checking your weight, a physical examination of the radiated area, and time to discuss the progress of your care. Your doctor may recommend a rest period during your therapy to allow time for your skin and surrounding tissues to recover from side effects such as skin reddening or muscle soreness. It is important to know that each treatment has its greatest effect one week after the radiation is given. Even if your skin looks just a little pink to you today, your doctor may want you to take a break based on his or her prediction of your future side effects. These breaks usually last only a few days and do not diminish the effectiveness of the overall treatment. A break can make you significantly more comfortable.

Radiation oncology treatments are often provided in basements because the shielding of the earth around the machines adds an extra level of safety. Unfortunately that means no windows can let light or sunshine in, and the treatment rooms are generally kept cool. If you are someone who dislikes the cold, dress warmly and bring along a sweater or a jacket. I found that my hot pink ski socks kept my feet and legs more comfortable—and they were a great conversation starter! Even after I changed into the hospital gown, I would slip on my jacket while waiting for my turn. You may want to add a warm hat if you happen to be bald or have very short hair during this time.

What do you think about while the radiation is being delivered to your tumor? It surprised me to learn that almost everyone I spoke to mentioned first, the sound of the door closing as the tech left the room, and second, the instinctive habit of counting while they listened to the whir of the machine. Other possibilities can offer a distraction, at least. At best, they may offer a way to enhance the effect of the treatment or your overall sanity through the process. If you are a person of faith, this is a great time to pray. It helped me to use visualization. I imagined that the invisible radiation was actually a beam of golden light, illuminating and healing every nook and cranny of my tissues. Some people see the radiation as a healing stream of water or a series of magic bullets that specifically target only cancer cells. Find the image that works best for you.

At home, your response to the radiation unfolds over the weeks. How can you stay most comfortable? These tips generalize to any part of the body that is treated with radiation.

- Make clothing choices that avoid elastic or seams on the treated area. For example, breast cancer patients may choose to avoid wearing a bra during these few weeks. A Softee is an undershirt-like garment that has sewn-in pockets for padding. It can get you through this relatively short time. Anything that rubs against your skin literally rubs away the outer layer of skin that protects you from raw skin, burns, or infections.

- Wear loose nightclothes that are non-binding in the area of treatment. Avoid sleeves or elastic waistbands that can rub.

- When you bathe, just let warm water flow over the area. Don't use soap and don't scrub or rub with a washcloth. When you dry off, just pat dry, don't rub.

- Use a moisturizer. Your radiation oncologist can give you one that protects the skin from dryness and itching. The comfort is worth the greasy feel. Ask before you put anything else on the affected skin because some chemicals can interfere with the effect of the radiation or irritate your skin, the last thing you need.

- The area radiated will be supersensitive to sunburn for the rest of your life, so cover up! Use sunscreen *always.*

- Fatigue is one of the most common side effects of radiation treatment. The loss of energy and general tiredness you may experience is different in character from the "tired" you feel after a workout or a long day outside. This fatigue is more chronic than acute and may persist even after a good night's sleep. The tiredness can strike without warning! I found myself feeling fine, then within minutes plummeting to exhaustion. Lying down for as little as fifteen minutes helped rejuvenate me so I could rejoin the day's activities. Frequent naps or rest periods can help you make the most of the energy you do have and can help your body heal. Generally you will begin to regain your energy within a couple of weeks after the end of your treatment. If you have an important event coming up, you may be able to use a one-time dose of Ritalin to give your energy a boost just for that event. Ask your doctor.

Although radiation therapy may be the easiest part of your treatment regimen physically, it is important to acknowledge that it does bring unique challenges. Fortunately because most of these challenges are emotional, you can do a lot to increase your level of comfort as you go along. As with any treatment, your attitude can be your best friend and can defuse potentially difficult times. How can you thrive while living your life around this schedule?

I strongly recommend taking the initiative in getting to know the people who will be providing your care. Introduce yourself. If you don't know someone's name or what they do, speak up. Say, "Hi! I'm Terry. I haven't met you yet. Who are you?" Then remember their name for next time. You will probably get a few startled looks, but you will have established that you are not just a case, not just a patient, but a *person* with a personality and a desire to communicate. If possible, reach out to shake a hand or ask for a helping hand to sit up after treatment. Make that tactile contact! Because the job of setting the machines can get pretty routine, you can add pleasure to both your own day and your technician's when you ask questions about his or her family, hobbies, or pets. The more you can become a friend to the person providing your care, the more cared for you will feel.

Someone who has "been there" and experienced the radiation treatment cycle can give moral support to the beginner. If you have a friend who has finished treatments, talk with him or her about what to expect. A great source of help and camaraderie can be found in the other patients who are undergoing therapy. Most people come on a daily basis, usually at the same time each day, so you may be seeing the same people for several weeks. If you are a newcomer, the old-timers will tell you, "You can do it!" When you have had several treatments, you will be the one offering encouragement to the folks just beginning. Sometimes there is a reluctance to speak to strangers in a waiting room. In this setting, however, you can help each other and discover something to look forward to—visiting with new friends. Once anyone breaks the code of silence with a "Hi" or "How's it going?" the conversation flows freely. It is a great relief to break out of isolation and become part of this new community, but it does take courage to make the first move.

Consider pampering your inner child, who may be pretty upset by all this indignity. I found that bringing along a small teddy bear to hold with my free hand helped a lot.

Sure, I'm a self-confident adult in most situations, but this isn't most situations and it is OK to be needy once in a while. You may prefer to bring a rabbit's foot, a small charm, or a photo, but whatever you choose, you are acting to preserve your sense of self.

My course of treatment was established at the beginning to be twenty-eight treatments, and I was not looking forward to the disruption of my daily life or the reminder of illness that treatments provided. I stopped in at a local candy store and hand-selected all of my favorite chocolates to be packaged in a one-pound box. I promised myself that this candy was only for use after each treatment and that I would reward myself for my perseverance with one piece each day. I counted the pieces, and knew that when the candy was half gone, I was halfway through. It was a great psychological boost. (Don't try this if you can't eat just one!) Maybe for you the daily treat can be a walk in the park or a phone call to a friend. Whatever you choose, this is another way of saying to yourself, "I am worth loving and nurturing."

In short:

- Take charge of your own emotional comfort during treatments by making personal, physical contact with the technicians and doctors who provide your care.

- Personalize the treatment experience with crazy hats or socks.

- Use imagery to visualize the healing effect of the radiation.

- Make clothing choices that are non-binding and non-rubbing.
- Bathe gently with no soap to the affected area, use a towel to blot dry, and apply a moisturizer.
- *Always* use sunscreen!
- Fatigue is common. Listen to your body. Rest as needed.
- Make friends with the other patients to raise everyone's level of comfort and cheer.
- Plan a daily "pat on the back" for yourself and a party when your treatments are over.

Complementary Care

The entire medical field is beginning to realize, or more accurately relearn, the truth that the human body, mind, and spirit are incredibly complex and intertwined. Anyone who wants to treat a disease or seek wellness must also consider the factors that influence health which are beyond the scope of conventional Western medical practice.

It is important to make a distinction between **alternative** treatments and **complementary** therapies. Proponents of **alternative** treatments advocate using them *in place of* conventional therapies. The difficulty is that scientific proof is lacking and often so are standards of licensing, training, and cleanliness. Sadly these potentially helpful therapies can easily be misused by unscrupulous providers more interested in their income than in your health. The biggest concern of all is that patients who could benefit greatly from standard medical care may delay that life-saving option in favor of treatments that could prove worthless. That delay can be deadly.

Complementary therapies are forms of treatment that are used *in conjunction with* conventional medicine. This kind of care includes yoga, massage, acupuncture, herbal remedies, hypnosis, special diets, and meditation. Many of these therapies can help significantly with your quality of life while you receive treatments such as surgery, chemotherapy, and radiation, and some have a measurable impact on your disease itself.

How do you choose when so much is unknown? How can you protect yourself from worthless treatments while not missing out on therapies that might help you? What follows is strictly my own opinion. For myself, I chose the most informed, up-to-date, and broadminded oncologist I could find. I evaluated his recommendations carefully, got second opinions, and did my own research. I fully agreed to the traditional treatment plan that was developed for me by my surgeon, radiation oncologist, and medical oncologist. This was the foundation of my healing path, and I evaluated every other option as something to consider *adding* to the treatments in progress. I personally believe that medical science offers a cancer patient the best chance of eradicating cancer. I also believe that other interventions for cancer patients, especially those which strengthen the immune system, can have a significant effect.

A great range of alternative treatment modalities are available. The National Center for Complementary and Alternative Medicine at the National Institutes of Health has divided the therapies into five categories: (1) alternative medical systems (homeopathic, naturopathic, traditional Chinese, and Ayurvedic medicine), (2) mind-body disciplines (meditation, prayer, mental healing, hypnosis, art, music and dance), (3) biological therapies (dietary supplements, herbal medicine), (4) manipulative and body-based therapies (chiropractic, osteopathic, and massage), and (5) energy therapies (Qigong, Reiki, therapeutic touch, pulse fields, and magnetic fields). An excellent resource that explores all of these is *Complementary and Alternative Medicine for Health Professionals* (see bibliography).

Alternative medical systems have been in use for hundreds, sometimes thousands, of years. Each has its own practitioners who are available in most cities.

Mind-body disciplines for cancer treatment include many forms of meditation, prayer, centering, and visualization. Often these recommend paying attention to your breathing. It can be difficult to "take a deep breath" during times of high stress or panic. A more helpful suggestion is to "exhale completely." Don't worry, the next breath will come in to that empty space. Creative pursuits such as writing, journaling, art, music, and dance are also mind-body interventions. Individuals often find a great deal of help on the cancer journey by choosing how to use their mind, awareness, and attitude in their best interest. So often the patient who gives up as soon as he receives his diagnosis does worse than the patient who decides to aggressively fight for his life. I am convinced that attitude makes a huge difference. It is the one factor we all have at our disposal, at no risk, for free.

Support groups are also included in the mind-body category. The scientific evidence about whether or not patients who participate in support groups actually live longer is still unclear. Support groups certainly have value, however, because the patients are able to deal with their disease more effectively along the way. This option may be more or less available to you, depending on your location. Many support services are now available on the Internet or social-media sites, and these can be a helpful alternative for those who are isolated. Be sure to use care choosing your site. The American Cancer Society and the National Cancer Institute are good places to start. One word of caution: If you feel worse after attending a support group meeting, it is probably not a good use of your time and energy. You might want to change groups or form your own. Some people are not comfortable with support groups and would rather confide in one or two other people who are dealing with similar challenges. It helps to talk to others who can reassure and encourage you along the way, but you are the best judge of what form that takes.

Dietary or supplement-based programs involve something you eat or take into your system, for example, by rubbing a compound onto your skin. The cancer section of your local bookstore offers many choices of "cancer prevention diets," most of which are based on anecdotal evidence or generalize from one specific fact to an entire diet plan. How do you know if a specific diet might help you, probably won't make any difference, or might harm you? You can protect yourself by asking these questions.

- Who recommends this diet and what are his or her qualifications? Is this a testimonial by an athlete or the result of a lifetime of study by a systematic researcher?

Is the book written by a physician, a layman, an entertainer, or a businessman?

- Who will profit from the sales of the book and the product? Be skeptical of programs that provide both the book and the dietary supplement.

- Is the recommended treatment so expensive or so restrictive that it is almost impossible to follow? If it is, the proponents will often blame failures on the patient rather than on their plan.

- Is the supplement safe? Might you be at risk because you are omitting any of the usual components of a healthy diet or because you may be overdosing on common vitamins or minerals?

- How long has the proposed plan been studied? Many dietary changes require a generation to determine safety and long-term effects.

- Do you know everything that is in the product? Prescription drugs contain carefully purified and accurately measured chemicals. Natural products such as herbal combinations usually contain a variety of ingredients (some yet to be identified) in addition to the one you hope will help you. **Just because a supplement is "natural" does not mean it is harmless!** It is a combination of tested and untested chemicals, some of which may actually be *harmful* to you. In addition, the purity and dose vary from manufacturer to manufacturer because no approval or regulation is required by the

Food and Drug Administration. It is critically important that nothing in your diet or supplements interacts with your prescription medications or chemotherapy agents. For example, soy products are often mentioned as a way to avoid the complications of menopause, but they mimic the effects of estrogen and may act similarly to worsen some kinds of hormone-sensitive cancers—the jury is still out. Be especially aware of the dangers of blood-thinning agents.

- Most important of all, what does your oncologist say? Her education, background, and life experience in dealing with cancer patients makes her uniquely qualified to advise you about the benefits or dangers of complementary products. Don't be reluctant to ask.

I can't leave this discussion without mentioning two excellent books, *Eating Well Through Cancer* and *The Cancer Fighting Kitchen* (see bibliography). Both provide practical recipes and suggest specific foods to eat or avoid if you have side effects such as constipation, diarrhea, or weight loss.

Manipulative and body-based therapies include overall fitness programs, individual exercise plans, acupuncture, massage, yoga, and others. These general wellness approaches are less likely than other interventions to have unexpected side effects. They have a long track record of safety—acupuncture has been used in Eastern cultures for thousands of years. These treatments increase your muscle tone and overall fitness, and they provide psychological benefits, too. You will need to increase activity gradually and slowly, staying alert to the response of your body to this new experience. Body work can make a big difference in your level of stress, muscle tension, posture, and overall sense of wellness. Because these treatments seldom interfere with or overlap with conventional medical treatments, they are less risky to add to your existing regimen than the more invasive biological therapies. As always, check with your doctor before you begin. Even if you do not affect the eventual outcome of your cancer battle, you will quite likely feel much better along the way, which is no small benefit!

Energy-based therapies work to manage the flow of energy through the body to improve wellness and minimize disease. The practitioner uses various hand manipulations to achieve a greater balance of energy flow.

You may have heard the term "integrative medicine." This refers to a combination of treatments from conventional medicine and complementary medicine which is considered safe and effective. Hospitals or cancer centers that embrace this approach believe that care for the whole person—body, mind, and spirit—leads to the best results. As our population ages, more and more places allow and encourage integrative medicine. Dr. Ralph Snyderman of Duke University says, "The integrative approach flips the health-care system on its head and puts the patient at the center, addressing not just symptoms, but the real causes of illness. It is care that is preventive, predictive, and personalized." Integrative care is in the middle of a spectrum with traditional care alone on one end and alternative care alone on the other end. Your care will usually be somewhere in between.

In short:

- The human body is incredibly complex and modern medicine does not have all the answers.

- State-of-the-art conventional medical care is the foundation of cancer treatment, but you can add many other interventions to increase your health.

- Biological programs involve something you eat or take into your system. Be extremely careful to avoid taking anything that can interact with your chemotherapy drugs. Be sure to let each of your doctors know everything you are taking: prescription, over-the-counter, or herbal preparations.

- Mind-body disciplines include yoga, acupressure, massage, and overall fitness programs.

- Mindfulness approaches include prayer, meditation, centering exercises, and visualization.

- To protect your health and your pocketbook, do a thorough investigation into the claims made by any program of alternative or complementary care, with special attention to possible conflicts of interest. Check out the credentials of the sponsors or proponents.

The Question of Pain

❧

Pain is a recurring theme throughout the cancer journey. Sometimes it is physical pain, the post-surgical acute sharp stabs that make you catch your breath. It may be minimal discomfort, tingling toes from neuropathy or achy muscles after radiation. A pervasive, non-specific pain in our hearts can come from the situation itself.

Remember your childhood? If you stubbed your toe or skinned your knee, it hurt. Someone loved it and bandaged it and you felt better. Suddenly pain is so complex! As cancer survivors, we may experience not only physical pain but also "soul pain." And the pain may come from many sources, not just an obvious physical cause. How do you proceed with this new challenge?

One of the most difficult dilemmas is uncertainty about when to seek help. I don't want to whine, but I also don't want to ignore important signals from my body. How do I know if that stiff knee or stitch in my side is the result of adhesions from prior surgery, growing older, overexertion, or a recurrence? When do I ask for professional opinions and when do I just wait and see? I think this is a really important question because the wondering itself results in "soul pain," the confusion and fear that can rob each day of the the joy we seek.

My personal answer to the "when to seek help" question is most unscientific: I listen to my gut feelings! If I notice discomfort or pain but I am fairly comfortable with waiting to see what happens next, I wait. Often the pain will resolve itself. If it does not, I will have more information to give to the doctor when I do talk to him or her. (Be prepared to answer these questions: How long has this been going on? What makes it better? Worse? Is it constant or intermittent?) Sometimes, however, I feel a pain that gets my immediate attention, and I know that I will not be at ease until it is checked out. I ask myself, "Why am I delaying seeking medical help?" If the answer is that I *might* be overreacting, I ask myself, "Is that so awful?" Then I make the phone call, explain the problem, and let the doctor decide what to do next. If you are delaying medical care because you have a sinking feeling in your stomach that this might be something serious (in other words, if you are afraid of bad news), then you should *certainly* call for a professional opinion! Delaying diagnosis of complications or recurrences only makes the problem more difficult to treat, and you will have lost valuable time. The days you wait will be tainted by fear, and you may feel remorse when you ask yourself, "Why didn't I call sooner?"

So what if the pain that worried you *is* caused by cancer? What if you cannot expect that things will gradually get better? How do you face the future?

First, be assured that pain management has come a long way in the last twenty years, and more breakthroughs are happening all the time. Much can be done to relieve pain, and doctors are much more aware of the importance of pain management for the quality of life for the whole person. Your doctor should be willing to discuss your pain levels with you and to provide whatever you need in terms of pain relief. If you begin taking a medication that does not work, be sure to speak up! Different kinds of pain respond to different painkillers, and the many different drugs available have different modes of action. Don't think that if your pain is unrelieved, you just have to "live with it." Ask for other alternatives. And ask if the dosage is the correct one for you—it may need to be adjusted. Pain medication can be administered in many different ways, so you can be assured that your need for pain relief can be addressed even if you are too ill to take medication by mouth.

Recent research shows that people who take pain medication to relieve pain (and not just to "feel good") rarely become addicted. As the pain decreases, so does their need for the medication. In fact, the latest research indicates that treating pain early, before it is overwhelming, results in both lower doses of medication per treatment and lower overall need for pain medication. The old myth that we need to "bear it as long as possible" is being replaced by new information which shows that pain which is relieved early is prevented from becoming overwhelmingly severe. Often, if one pain medication is not enough, a combination of drugs and dosage schedules can bring you the comfort you need.

Just a note: Sometimes the pain is relieved by medication, but the side effects can be most uncomfortable. Many pain medications, especially narcotics, cause upset stomach or constipation. Fortunately these side effects can be treated or avoided. You can often avoid stomach upset by modifying the time the medicine is taken. Ask whether it should be taken on an empty stomach or with food. Constipation can be a serious and miserable condition, but it is avoidable and treatable. The sooner it is addressed, the better. Be sure to let your doctor know if this is a concern for you. As the first line of defense, drink lots of water. Regular exercise such as walking helps keep things moving. You may need to take additional preparations to soften your stools or to promote regularity. This is not a do-it-yourself project, however. Be sure to work with your physician so your overall medication needs can be addressed together.

In addition to pain relief medications, pain can be addressed through techniques that focus on how your mind processes your pain. Stress, anxiety and muscle tension result in both increased pain and decreased ability to handle that pain. Relaxation and use of imagery may help. Hypnosis can be a valuable tool for both stress reduction and pain relief by working with the unconscious mind to override conscious pain responses and allow for increased calm and peace, both physically and mentally.

What about "soul pain"? This may not be the most accurate name for the condition, but I think most of us have experienced it. The primary pain problem we face may not be physical but emotional, spiritual, or psychological. However you describe it, as human beings we share an awareness of a kind of fundamental unrest, a central disordering of our world, a profound shifting in point of view as a result of our cancer diagnosis. I believe this loss of innocence, the realization that we are mortal people in an imperfect body, can be the most challenging part of our growth into fully developed people. It is difficult to face this new reality of a body (and perhaps a spirit, too) that is "broken." Because soul pain is intangible, we are tempted to hope it will just go away. "Maybe tomorrow will be brighter," you think. But if ignored, soul pain can lead to depression and more misery. It is worth the struggle of working through the difficulty to come to some resolution and peace.

Soul pain can result from a variety of sources, just as a painful foot can result from sunburn, a stubbed toe, arthritis, or too-tight shoes. Obviously the key to relieving this kind of pain is to identify the cause as precisely as possible. Simply knowing the source of the pain will often allow you to see how to relieve it. As you read on, just disregard the pain problems that do not apply to you. Use what is helpful as a starting point for your own exploration of your inner space.

The most obvious soul pain is based in fear (see Chapters 1 and 3). Fear is most directly addressed by being as precise as possible about the exact kind of fear you have.

Do you fear pain? Social ostracism? Being different? Being dead? The dying process? Isolation? All of the above? The fears that any one person suffers are impacted by your prior experience, so the intensity and character of the fear is unique to you. Because the fear is specific to you, you can find the solution to the fear that will work for you. For example, if your fear is isolation, you can take concrete steps to reach out for the company of friends with phone calls or e-mails. If your main fear is physical pain, you can do research into the huge array of medications and biofeedback techniques now available to treat pain.

Another kind of soul pain which is less obvious, and yet perhaps even more important, is the pain of concern about your relationship with God—the question of eternity. Whatever your faith background, facing death will bring you to consider the profound question of "What next?" If you are a believer you may be even more unwilling to question the future than a person with no religious affiliation because you may think your religion defines for you a set of teachings about the afterlife which you must accept as your own. In reality, however, each one of us must come to grips with this fundamental unknown ourselves, in our own heart of hearts. We may never know the answers until we are there, but it is crucially important to ask the questions. Otherwise, this major piece of unfinished business can eat away at our peace of mind, lurking at the edge of our consciousness until it is addressed. This time of illness and soul pain provides an invitation to explore our own faith or perhaps to gather information about other world views or religions. Ultimately our questions can lead us to the peace of heart that comes from trusting God, no matter what challenges face us.

Sometimes the major source of emotional pain is our concern for those we love. How does my illness affect them? Am I robbing my children of their childhood, of their future security, of their parent? Am I spending too much money on medical bills and placing my family in great financial need? How will my spouse deal with both a job and the demands of running the household when I can't help out? What will my family do without me? I want to be here to hold my grandchildren! This relational pain is real. It can be put in perspective, however, by recognizing that it exists. It was a revelation to me to discover that those I love have far more resilience, maturity and coping ability than I gave them credit for. In fact, as I learned to express my concerns openly, I marveled at the way each of us grew. In every single case, an honest expression of my concerns and sorrow resulted in relief of pain for both parties. The greatest pain is to keep your worries under wraps, concealed, to "protect" others. The result of that dishonesty is that your child or spouse will have to imagine what is troubling you and will not understand your real feelings. It takes a lot of courage, but taking the plunge to say what is in your heart can heal you both.

If you find that your pain revolves around unfinished parenting or worry about a spouse's future, you can find ways to be a part of the future. I know women who have purchased birthday cards for their children for many years into the future and written age-appropriate motherly advice for their beloved children to receive even after the death of their mom. I wrote notes to be given to my children on the occasion of their weddings, just because it is so important to me to be sure that they will know of my love and concern. If I am hit by a car tomorrow, my message will be preserved for them. It is also possible to make voice recordings of music or loving thoughts. This pain of unfinished business can be addressed, and to do so frees you to enjoy the life you share *now*.

In short:

- Call your doctor when you have a gut feeling that a pain may represent a serious change in your body.

- Don't avoid taking pain medication because you worry about addiction.

- Treating pain early can result in less total medication needed.

- Exercise and drink lots of water to avoid constipation, a common and avoidable source of pain.

- Recognize that some pain, soul pain, needs to be acknowledged, examined, and dealt with to allow you to heal it.

Living with Recurrences (Read Part II!)

❧

From the moment of the first cancer diagnosis, the ever-present drumbeat in the mind is, "What if it comes back?" This cancer awareness is so constant that it seems that no matter what else is happening in the world outside, each book, conversation, movie, or business transaction is completed in spite of the distraction of the cancer chant inside the head. It seemed to me that I would never be able to forget that I had been a cancer patient, never be able to spend time "free," to live completely focused on the present without my cancer filter. As time went by, weeks and months, I began to notice periods of five or ten minutes when I felt like my old self, times when I became absorbed in a present reality that did not include my illness. As the months stretched into years, whole days would pass when I didn't think of cancer even once. The passage of time *does* heal the raw places in our sense of identity caused by cancer. I believe, though, that once you have experienced a full dose of the cancer reality, you never completely escape from the "what if's." For me, the most scary "what if" is, "What if it comes back?"

About two years after my initial diagnosis with ovarian cancer I was diagnosed with breast cancer. Of course, I was overwhelmed and stunned, but my reaction was tempered by the knowledge that I was stronger emotionally and spiritually than I had been at my first diagnosis. I had a number of effective coping mechanisms to help me through the next adventure.

The most helpful insight was realizing that I had done much of the work necessary to live fully in each moment. I understood and believed that I would someday die, like everyone else. I realized that nothing at all I could do would ensure that I would live forever. I knew that what mattered more than the length of my life was what I chose to do with the time I was given. My eyes were open to the reality that no life is without challenges and that I can be joyful in spite of illness.

Hope. This is an active verb, a positive choice each of us can make in the face of whatever comes our way. No one can see the future, and no one can tell you that you have six months to live. A doctor may be able to say that the last person they saw with your condition lived six months, but that is very different from saying that *you* will live only six months. Our bodies and our world are in a constant state of change. New discoveries are being made each day, and refinements of old treatments can bring better results with fewer side effects. Research continues to explore novel approaches to this disease, from genetic engineering to transplants to immune system drugs. Ongoing clinical trials of new drugs and therapies abound. And there are always the surprising few patients who recover with no explanation, against all odds (see bibliography, *Radical Remission*). Many people become cancer-free after treatment for recurrence and live a normal life span. If you operate from a position of hope, you look for the ways you can be one of them! You choose to believe that you will benefit from whatever comes your way physically, emotionally, or spiritually. Hope sends your body the message that it is valued and sends your mind and heart the message that you can still contribute to the rest of humanity, even if only with your love. Hope nurtures an attitude that is healthy for you because it causes you to focus on what is right, on what you *can* do, and not on what you lack.

Remember. Go back in your mind over the last treatments you had, and recognize yes, the treatments might have been difficult. Then remind yourself that you *did* bear them, and you can bear them again if you choose. Consider how much you have grown in resourcefulness, patience, and compassion and realize that still more growth is possible. Enter into the process—don't passively assume that you can never be happy again. "Happy" has a way of being redefined according to the challenges of our lives. I can remember being blissfully happy when I was finally allowed to take a bath following surgery!

Give. Nothing brings meaning to our lives as much as the awareness that we have something to contribute. Maybe you will never assume the role of president of the corporation again, but that doesn't mean that you have nothing to give. Be an encourager. Give love to all you meet. Now that you have time to consider what causes you support, give to charities. Give your listening ear to others who can profit from the wisdom you have acquired. I'll never forget Joe, a leukemia patient who came in daily for treatments at the infusion center where I received my chemotherapy. Everyone knew Joe and everyone loved Joe. He never complained. Instead, he reached out to every other person he met with a bubbling enthusiasm and interest in them with the assumption that they were valuable and interesting people. He lived his life to the brim and gave more during his cancer years than he ever could have in a typical giving profession. Be a giver, not a taker.

Plan. Look ahead to the opportunities that await you—a son's graduation from high school, a granddaughter's wedding, or a special trip. Be eager for the joys that are ahead. How sad it is to die before we die because we fear the disappointment that may come if we anticipate events that we cannot share. Look ahead with enthusiasm, but allow for last-minute changes in plans if necessary. If you are having a good day on the day of the celebration, not only will the activity be a joy but you will also have savored the delight of anticipation.

I love this quote from George Bernard Shaw. "My life belongs to the whole community, and as long as I live, it is my privilege to do for it whatsoever I can. I want to be thoroughly used up when I die, for the harder I work, the more I live. Life is no 'brief candle' to me. It is a sort of splendid torch, which I have got hold of for the moment, and I want to make it burn as brightly as possible before handing it on to future generations."

In short:

- Remember that many people live with recurrent cancer and still find great fulfillment.

- Choose to be hopeful.

- Remind yourself that you have come through treatments before and can again.

- Many people become cancer-free after treatment for a recurrence.

- Give whatever you can to those around you—a smile, a caring word, a hug.

- Plan for the future.

- Keep living each today.

Long-term Effects
(Staying Well)

⚜

What about this body of yours, the one that went through the surgery or chemotherapy or radiation, or all three, maybe repeatedly? Your body will never be the same, but it can be pretty good! You will, however, have some definite limitations to keep in mind from this point on.

After your cancer treatment has ended, you will still need to be checked out regularly by your doctor. This is considered routine surveillance. You will still need to be screened for second primary cancers, for instance, by continuing with recommended mammograms or colonoscopies. It is important to manage long-term and late effects of disease and treatment. Of course you want to do your best to stay healthy with good living habits. You also need to be your own advocate by making sure your care is coordinated between all of your doctors. Everyone needs to stay informed.

As always, the best course of action is to ask your doctors for their recommendations about limits on your activities. One area of concern may be your ability to lift weights. You may have to be careful about normal activities of daily living, carrying babies or grocery bags. In addition, be sure to get advice before beginning any exercise regimen.

If your cancer treatment required surgery, you may be dealing with several complications from the surgery itself. Sometimes the disruption of tissues during surgery results in "over-healing" with the kind of scarring called keloids. These harmless, raised bumpy areas can occur anywhere and can be unsightly (although they are harmless). If they bother you, you can have the scar revised with another surgical procedure to remove this excess scar tissue. This is only a matter of appearance, not a health issue.

Surgery can also result in internal scar tissue formation. In the abdomen or elsewhere, this scarring can take the form of adhesions, which are fibrous connections between organs or parts of organs that normally slide easily past each other. Imagine someone using superglue to connect one part of your small intestine to another! If the adhesions form a ring around your intestines, you may develop a bowel obstruction, a blockage of the intestinal tract. A bowel obstruction is a surgical emergency and a condition to take very seriously. Any change in bowel habits, persistent or increasing pain, nausea or vomiting, are messages from your body that should not be ignored. Prompt medical attention can usually relieve this condition.

Scarring can also lead to decreased mobility. It is really important to continue stretching exercises for life—a few minutes a day can maintain your range of motion. It's true: Use it or lose it!

Another possible result of surgery, radiation, or both is disruption of the lymphatic system. The lymphatic system is a means for the body to fight infection. Normally the fluids in the system pass freely and easily from your hand to your armpit or your foot to your groin. In areas that have been injured, and especially in areas where lymph nodes have been removed for diagnostic purposes, the free flow of lymph fluid can become blocked. If this blockage is significant, you may experience lymphedema, which is a swelling, usually of an extremity, resulting from the accumulation of lymphatic fluid. Sometimes the risk may not be mentioned by your surgeon or radiation oncologist. It doesn't affect every patient and it is unpredictable who will be affected. It is a good idea to ask your doctor if you might experience problems with lymphedema and what precautions he or she suggests. Prevention can be fairly straightforward and well worth your time and energy. Lymphedema can occur at any time after radiation or surgery, even years later. This condition can be serious, and if untreated it can progress from a little swelling to a great deal of swelling. If you notice tight rings, swollen ankles, puffy skin, or a feeling of heaviness, ask your doctor if you have lymphedema. Several alternatives can help resolve the problem, from pressure bandages to special stroking massages. The condition can be uncomfortable and inconvenient by itself. Of even greater concern, however, is the risk of cellulitis, a breakdown of the tissues in the affected area, characterized by pain and redness. Cellulitis is most often treated with antibiotics because it also puts you at risk of an infection in a much larger area. Be sure to call your doctor if you discover any areas that might be infected. Act quickly! If some of your lymph nodes have been removed, your risk of a serious and fast-moving infection is much greater than it was before your cancer treatments. You will need to be vigilant.

Whether or not you have lymphedema, you need to be especially careful to avoid injury to any area treated with surgery or radiation. For example, if you are a breast cancer survivor, you will want to avoid any break in the skin on the affected side or any constriction of that arm. This means you need to be sure that you ask your health-care providers to use your non-affected arm for blood tests, for shots, for IVs, or for blood pressure checks. Do not wear any accessory (ring, watch, or bracelet) that is binding. Avoid elastic that is tight enough to restrict blood flow. Make it a matter of habit to wear protective gloves whenever you are at risk for scratches or punctures, for instance, when you are pruning the roses or pulling weeds. It is also important that manicures be done gently, with minimum disruption of the skin or nail bed.

Speaking of infections, you need to be aware that some cancer treatments can result in an increased vulnerability to infection from any source. You may have persistent fatigue, for instance, or a chronically low white blood cell count. (The white blood cells normally protect us from infection.) It just makes sense to take extra precautions such as getting a yearly flu shot or protective immunizations if you travel. If you visit other countries, follow the advice for preventing "traveler's diarrhea." Drink only bottled water or beverages (no ice cubes) and avoid fresh, uncooked fruits and vegetables. Your oncologist may even prescribe antibiotics to take along on the trip, just in case.

If you were treated with chemotherapy you might experience "chemo brain" (see Part II, Chapter 23). Another possible long-term effect is neuropathy. Chemotherapy-induced peripheral neuropathy can interfere with sensation and movement in the hands and arms, feet and legs, or bladder and bowel. Neuropathy doesn't cause weakness but can affect balance and gait. Rehabilitation efforts focused on improving balance can help; some medications can bring significant relief. Ask your doctor about those tingling hands and feet.

You need to be constantly careful about sun protection, especially if you have had radiation therapy. The skin in the area of treatment will burn more quickly and easily than normal surrounding skin. Be sure to use a high SPF sunscreen, wear protective clothing, seek shade, and avoid sun exposure during the heat of the day.

Your doctors can tell you what follow-up is needed for your kind of cancer. Maybe you'll be released entirely, with only normal checkups suggested. More often, your surgeon, internist, oncologist and/or radiation oncologist will want to re-examine you at intervals ranging from weeks to years. Often a physical examination is augmented by laboratory studies, such as blood tests, to be sure no delayed effects from your treatment are showing up. An X-ray of the area in question or repeat CT scans may be ordered. This extra watchfulness can help catch potential problems before you experience any symptoms.

By now you are an expert at listening to your body's messages, and your personal alertness is an important tool. If you see any changes get them checked out right away, even if it means calling or returning to your doctor before your regularly scheduled appointment.

As a matter of prudence it is a good idea to keep your own personal copy of your medical information. Your chart may be far too extensive to copy. (I'm working on Volume Two at my oncologist's office.) The critical information you should have at hand, in case you move or your doctors do, is much more manageable. You need copies of any surgery "op report," pathology reports from biopsy or tumor-removal surgery, X-ray or CT reports, and the treatment plan or summary of treatments given by the oncologist and/or radiation oncologist. This includes chemotherapeutic agents given, number of treatments and dosage, and the number of radiation therapy treatments, the total radiation given, and the localization. Once you have these documents put them away as an insurance policy in case of future need. I have a "cancer cupboard" in which I store medical records, my wig, scarves, and books. I close the door and am elated at my current wellness.

In short:

- Your new emotional and spiritual insights go along with

a body that requires loving attention.

- Be aware of surgery scars and watch for signs of trouble from bowel obstruction or limited range of motion.

- Watch for swelling, especially in the extremities, which can indicate lymphedema or infection.

- Use preventative medicine wisely. Get that flu shot! Be extra careful when you travel.

- Use sunscreen always, especially on skin that has been exposed to radiation or is scarred.

- See your doctors for follow-up checkups as recommended, even if you are feeling fine.

- Listen to your body for feedback and investigate any changes.

- Keep a personal copy of your medical history.

No Evidence of Disease (NED)

⚜

So you have made it! You have successfully navigated the journey we call cancer. What next? Naturally you have great reason to rejoice each and every day of your new life that you are, quite simply, alive. But you are not the same "you" that started on this journey, weeks or months or years ago. You are now a cancer survivor in a special sense, a person who is clinically free of evidence of cancer. How are you different?

Certainly your emotional and spiritual insights will be a part of you from this point on. You have a new sense of priorities and a new awareness of both your powerlessness and your courage. You have confronted some choices you would not have believed you could survive—but you did. You have a new sense of confidence and a greatly decreased need for the approval of others. You have been tried and have dug deep for the resources to see you through. Congratulations!

I rejoice that *right now* I am well. I savor the moment and relish the health I enjoy. When I was diagnosed, I asked myself what I could learn from the experience of dealing with cancer, what the specific lesson was for me. The lesson?

Life is the adventure! Life is not on hold while I am ill—life is whatever the day brings and whatever I bring to the day. I discovered depths of pain, fear, and sorrow I could not imagine—and heights of wellness, faith, and joy I would never have believed possible. I learned to enjoy each today, fully aware that my days are limited in number.

When I was the sickest—most discouraged, most alone, and least capable of doing—I learned that at its core, life is meaningful because of love. No matter how sick I got, I could *still* give and receive love, constantly. This fundamental truth transformed me.

You will have discovered truths along the way, too. Truth is so much more than one person can absorb. I think of the poem I learned in grammar school about the blind men and the elephant. One touched the tail and said an elephant is like a rope. Another bumped against the side and thought an elephant is like a wall. The one who touched the ear thought it like a fan, and the one who touched the trunk said it is like a snake. Of course we know that each of them had "seen" only a part of the animal.

Life, illness, and wellness will always remain mysterious. The *whole* truth is as elusive to us as that elephant was to the blind men. But each one of us must search for the portion of the truth that we *can* see and know. Our search for meaning frees us to celebrate life!

PART II

I'm Having a Good Run of Days

Introduction

Part II, *I'm Having a Good Run of Days*, has been on my mind since I wrote my first book, *Cancer: The Adventure of Your Life* (which appears here as Part I). Where did I get the title? A dear friend was dealing with three different, long-term cancers for several years, along with plenty of side effects, a colostomy, and cellulitis. She was in and out of treatment and the hospital. Whenever I saw her, I would ask how she was doing. Her answer never varied: "I'm having a good run of days." Because that is how she perceived her life, that is how she *lived* her life, with gratitude and gusto.

I hope Part II will help you heal. What is "healing"? It isn't the same as "cure." Cure refers to the whole body being free of cancer. It's a doctor construct based on scans and numbers, a passive reflection of what has been *done to you*. Healing, on the other hand, does not necessarily refer to the absence of cancer. Healing is the recognition that *what I do*, actively, can allow me to recognize the gift of the day, the joy of interacting with others and fullness of life right now. I listen to my body and that allows me to care for others on a different level, at the soul, the place of peace and healing. Spiritual healing isn't restoring us to a place we used to be, but rather getting rid of the blocks we have acquired that prevent us from listening to our souls which have always been within us. We can listen to the wisdom of God.

I have grown in wisdom as a result of walking with hundreds of cancer patients, both those who will be cured and those who live with cancer as a chronic condition. I have been blessed to know many people whose cancer was a constant companion for many years. Some eventually died, but others continue to be an inspiration to me. The lessons I have learned apply to cancer patients; however, anyone who is dealing with a life-threatening illness will find food for thought here. My goal for Part II is to give encouragement to those who are further along their journey. A different intensity of challenge exists for people who are facing the reality that their cancer may never go away completely. It is a quantum leap in thinking, similar to the one that happens when you hear the words, "You have cancer." Your world shifts, your priorities change. It can feel very lonely and scary. I hope to ease your worries so that you can spend your time and energy on loving life, not re-inventing the wheel.

Although I am a twenty-three-year survivor of ovarian cancer and a twenty-year survivor of two different breast cancers, I am blessed to be free of cancer as I write. I *don't* know from my own experience how you feel—no one can know that but you! Many of the insights that follow are based on conversations with people I greatly admire who face their diagnosis with both hope and courage. I interviewed people who are living with cancer and asked for their wisdom at this stage of their journey. Some of their quotes are included here, with their permission.

As with Part I, each chapter can be read independently of the others. Some topics will interest you now. Some may not apply to your situation. Feel free to skip those.

If you are reading this, you are alive. You are already a survivor! The way you face your future is up to you.

Wisdom From Those Walking the Journey

❧❦❧

As I looked over the comments of patients I interviewed I was struck by the many threads of agreement in point of view and attitude. It's a good place to start: hearing the wisdom of others. I quote them directly. Some of the comments may resonate with you. You are not alone!

Most folks were passionate when I asked, "What would you tell people *not* to say or do?" Here are their responses.

What was **unhelpful** to you?

"Don't say, 'You are strong and can lick this like other cancer patients have.' The speaker means well but doesn't understand that all cancers are not the same."

"Don't argue about the beliefs of the patient. Especially don't challenge or try to change their faith beliefs. You may not agree with the patient, but do not use this illness as a chance to 'convert' them."

"Don't have a 'last' event, whatever it is! Don't talk about last visits, last concerts, last holiday meals. To declare something as "last" implies divine knowledge we don't have. I found myself having a 'living wake' for months. I felt like I should have been in a casket with people throwing flowers on me!"

"Don't say, 'You poor thing!' (I'd rather hear, 'You're doing great!')"

"Don't refer to treatments as 'grueling."

"Don't say, 'We're poisoning your system.'"

"Don't even *think* of me as a damaged person. I can tell from your body language what you are thinking."

What was **helpful** to you?

"Think of me as a whole person."

"Forget that I have cancer. I am still me."

"Help me with chores and meals!"

"Visits are a wonderful diversion and a great way to stay involved in the lives of people I love."

"Let's act like I don't have cancer and just relax and behave exactly as we used to. I don't need pity or seek it. I won't be as fast or as strong as I was, but I will do what I can. We can accomplish whatever we want; I want to participate."

"Ask them to pray and be supportive of me as my disease progresses with its many challenges."

How do you handle a difficult day? What are your **coping tips?**

"On awakening, I say to myself, 'This is going to be a good day! I woke up on the right side of the dirt!'"

"My caregiver has a tougher time than I do!"

"I try to live just one minute, one hour at a time during the day. I have learned each day is a precious gift to be used to its fullest, whether I'm totally incapacitated or somewhat active."

"I have low-energy days when I can't get much done. I go and do what I can and then rest. Then I go out and do something else until I need to rest again. I have come to realize that if I'm still breathing, I'm alive. If I'm alive, then I'm living. When I can't draw my next breath I will think I'm dying, and not a moment before. I breathe deep and don't panic!"

"In general, what helps most is to have as much normalcy as possible. Even on a 'low' day I go out with my friends. I make a date and spend a social event free of 'cancer talk.'"

"I only have to get through one day—today. I've managed this far. God has been good to me. I have a lot of people praying for me. My treatments (and the prayers) will help the way they are supposed to."

"I have cancer! I back off and try to make things easier for myself rather than push through. I am a lot more gentle with myself. Now if I don't want to do something, I don't."

How has cancer changed your **relationships**?

"I am more patient, both with myself and with others."

"I love staying connected—but in person, not electronically! I need the body language and back-and-forth conversation. I appreciate my family for all they do, and I have come to learn how to accept help. I have more empathy with people who are grumpy."

"My real friends are closer now. We have an understanding of how important we are to each other. I never realized that my friends loved me in the past. Now it's obvious. We have achieved a new level of honesty."

"Staying in touch with family and friends is most encouraging. This is a priority no matter how bad I feel."

What have been the **blessings** of this disease for you and for those who love you? (Some of the most encouraging answers of all were to this question.)

"Tolerance, patience, and an active relationship with God are some of my blessings."

"I have been able to connect on a deeper level with friends and family. We don't talk about nonsense and avoid the real issues anymore."

"I found out that strangers are kinder than I expected. I have received help from perfect strangers in all kinds of situations and places."

"I have come to see how giving, generous, loving, and thoughtful people are. I understand that sometimes people don't feel good, and I have more empathy."

"I'm a lot more considerate. I don't take things for granted. I am more appreciative."

What are your overall comments on "the **journey**"?

"Don't *expect* a miracle, but *believe* in them! Feel the prayers of others."

"Everybody should think about death; we're all going to die! We should *all* live as if we don't know how long we have to live—none of us knows. This is *my* journey; I accept it."

"My favorite quote is from Oprah Winfrey. 'Doing the best at this moment puts you in the best place for the next moment.'"

"A deep burning will to live and having a more positive outlook is helping with the disease and quality of my life."

"I take solace in knowing that while my story has a tragic ending, I can write good chapters in the meantime. Knowing the ending doesn't mean you know the story. The ending is only loosely pertinent to the current chapter."

"I'm in a rush. I think that living with intensity will allow me to cover more ground quickly. I'm also trying to deflect stress. Most of the things I used to stress over don't seem as important compared to a life and death struggle."

"I did say goodbye to all of my friends. I didn't want to pass away without having contacted the important people from my life. Some have come across the country and the state to visit. I wanted to let them know how important they were to me and how much I appreciated their friendship. I am free to go at any time now, without regrets."

"I'm actually in 'slowed down mode,' but I know lifetime care will be necessary. I'd like to think that I'm exceptionally tough and will prove the experts wrong. I'd like to think that I can drive rogue cells right out of my body. I try to stay open to healing. I also try not to fool myself, so I continue to proceed as though I only have a couple of years left."

"It feels good to be my authentic self without masks. I felt like I had been the person I was expected to be long enough. I have a couple of years to be my genuine self without apologies. Like it or leave it, this is who I really am and you are free to shun me if you need to. In fact, if I'm not acceptable to someone, we need to part anyway."

"I wanted to model courage and perseverance in the face of extreme adversity. I exceeded the expectations of everyone."

Each of us has our own experience of coming to "healing." Your experience will be your own, not necessarily like anyone else's.

One friend wanted to share her own insights as her legacy. She said,

"My doctors and I agree that healing follows belief. There are Teachers who have come into the flesh, Jesus and others, who showed us the full potential of humans and taught miracles. The Teachers taught us how to use our own healing capacities. I believe they came to show us how to heal, not just by working on physical needs but also by showing us we have so much spiritual potential that has been stolen from us. We have been 'dumbed down' to consider only the material and scientific. We *are* fully able to realize the potential of all of our Teachers. We *must* believe in our own full potential as human beings. As a culture, we have lost that awareness and that must be our next exploration. It is the person who is his *own* healer, not the doctor or another person. Children know this until we teach them otherwise.

"Healing follows belief. You need to work in and cultivate the spiritual realm. Move into the feeling of what it would be to be *well* in your situation. Embrace it with your whole being and thoughts. As you embody the experience in your mind of seeing yourself well, running or biking, as you feel your whole body responding to this message, your body embraces the experience. Our spiritual self is the huge bottom of the iceberg that we don't see. Allopathic medicine isn't fully aware of, and doesn't yet embrace, spiritual or nutritional components of healing. Too often the message is 'the doctor will do it,' not that the patient heals himself. The healer is within."

An artist friend, a retired doctor and Al-Anon member, used his painting as a way to process the impact of his diagnosis on his life.

"Before diagnosis, I painted myself as separate, intact, sheltered from the chaos around me. At the time of my diagnosis I dissolved, really, and merged with the chaos. My delusional armor of health was lost and I felt like I wiped out all my thoughts of the future. As time passed, my attachment to who I was started to lessen. My energy was comforted with spiritual awareness. Over time, I was able to return again to my belief in my Higher Power—the energy around me. When you are at this level of soul-consciousness, you can see the suffering around you and be an instrument to help others come to a place of serenity.

"As medical professionals, we can get lost in thinking that our caring for other people, *about* them, must be diminished in order to work effectively; that we must be detached. As cancer patients, we are empowered to extend care on a level that is personal. We can be fully present with the suffering of another patient in a more complete way. We learn the need to ask for help for ourselves. In turn, we can share with other patients the care we received, to encourage them to *accept* help from God and from others.

"I came to believe that I am supposed to be here. I will always be one breath away from death. I have come to see death not as an enemy but as a friend. I think we get cancer to raise our consciousness and awareness of who we really are. Cancer gives us an opportunity to meet with our true self before we die."

Another dear friend, given a diagnosis of stage 4 pancreatic cancer, said, "What am I supposed to do with THIS?" Her answer can apply to us all. "Let your light so shine before men that they may see the good that you do and give glory to God." Her mantra became, "Let your light shine."

In short:

- Patients facing a future that includes cancer will learn how others can be helpful or unhelpful to them.

- Patients can discover personal coping abilities that make the journey easier and more meaningful.

- Blessings can and do appear at any stage of the journey.

Components of Wellness
With Cancer

Where to begin? Our health is such an interrelated puzzle. If everything affects everything else, how can we develop strategies to come to optimum health?

The four components of wellness are physical, mental, emotional, and spiritual. All are necessary. At any given time, one or another may seem to be more critical; but overall, each must be addressed in order to achieve maximum wellness. I'd like to explore them one at a time, since each presents its own challenges in the cancer journey.

The primary concern of the physicians, nurses, and health professionals is the **physical** component. They are pros at treating the symptoms of the disease. They do so every day, and they have an awesome arsenal of tools to treat that aching back, that swollen arm, that infected wound. Let's take it as a given that you are receiving state-of-the-art medical care from terrific doctors and nurses, and your care of the physical parts of the illness is going fine.

It's interesting to note that when the doctor asks you, "How are things going?" he or she is really asking, "Do you have a fever? Is anything hurting that wasn't hurting before? Do you have a new rash?" If you don't report a new "symptom" and your "numbers," those all-important lab results, are within the expected range, the doctor may say, "You're doing just *fine!*"

Actually that may be news to you, when you feel anything but fine. You may feel pretty bad, in fact! But too many patients are reluctant to rock the boat and point out the "little" things that are bothering them in the physical realm. These things, little from the point of view of the doctor or nurse, are often very large in the view of the patient and the caregiver for whom they can be a major source of distress.

I would like to mention four. The first is insomnia. Not every doctor will ask, "How are you sleeping?" Some think that if you don't say anything, you must be sleeping just fine. Some doctors think that no one sleeps very well, and if they don't ask, they don't have to deal with it! Most are just too focused on eradicating a tumor to worry about the little things, like comfort! It is up to you (or your caregiver if you are reluctant) to point out that you are exhausted all the time because you are having a terrible time going to sleep at night. Fortunately help is available. Behavioral modifications can make a huge difference—a bedtime routine, an earlier evening meal, a warm bath, relaxing music, avoiding stress in the evening, and going to bed only when you are sleepy. Often exercise during the day (not at bedtime) can reset your energy cycles so that you are more inclined to be sleepy at night. Meditation and yoga can be helpful for setting up a more relaxed you overall.

If you have tried these things and are still suffering from long and sleepless nights, speak up! Your doctor won't know this is a problem unless you say so. Many medications, both over-the-counter and prescription, can help. No one wants to be dependent on a sleep aid, but not sleeping is bad for your health and your coping ability the next day. This is a long-term effort, and you need to be able to choose wisely for optimum health. Some of the prescription medications can be used as needed and the dosage reduced as you become more able to set up a sleep routine. Be assured that sleep disturbances are often a part of the journey through cancer and you are not alone.

The second physical dilemma is pain control. Recent research has shown that controlling pain is much more easily done with greater effect, shorter duration, and less medication, if the control begins early. Our nervous system pathways are similar to tracks in the snow—the first time a track is made, it is fairly superficial and easy to erase. The more that track is trampled, the deeper the ruts and the easier it is for future trackers to follow the same path. Decide that you can and will control your pain early on while the path is still just superficial, rather than waiting until the ruts are deep indeed and your nerves automatically follow the same pain path. This is true for any kind of pain, no matter the source—treating it early and effectively is always the best option, not only for now but for your future.

Many patients think pain is inevitable and that they are whining if they tell their doctor that their pain medication is inadequate. It's true that our lives may never be pain-free but it is almost always possible to manage pain. The newest pain medications can be effective beyond what was possible just a few years ago. Pain medications work through a variety of different mechanisms and each class of drugs acts on the pain in different ways. Some actually work on the source of the pain. Some tell the brain not to respond with a "distress" signal. Some work on the overall perception of pain. The point is, there are many ways to approach this problem. If you are still in pain in spite of the medications you have been prescribed, be sure to tell your doctor. He or she can modify the dose, change medications, or suggest combinations of drugs that may increase their effectiveness. A huge range of complementary treatments can bring pain relief. Many chronic pain sufferers find that yoga, tai chi, acupuncture, stretches, Reiki, or massage can improve not only the specific site of the pain, but can also provide fitness, freedom of movement, relaxation, and stress reduction. Many of these techniques have been used for thousands of years and are safe and effective.

Just a note. Any change in pain medication can have unintended effects on other parts of your interconnected body. One of the most common side effects is constipation. Drugs can cause respiratory difficulty, a "spacey" feeling, or sleepiness. Some exceptionally effective drugs can also cause hallucinations or difficulty in thinking that can be pretty profound. Many of these side effects can be treated by dietary changes or behavior changes to assist coping and remembering. In every case you and your doctor will need to determine the "risk versus benefit" ratio. If the pain is so debilitating that you cannot function, you might be willing to accept increased sleepiness. If the pain is tolerable but still noticable, you might choose to live with that bit of pain or to treat it more conservatively. You can decide day to day what is needed for your comfort and can change your mind as needed. Taking pain medication is NOT a sign of weakness; it is doing the best you can to live a meaningful, full life right now and into the future.

The third physical symptom that can escape detection is depression, anxiety, or fear. Physical issues and emotional ones overlap, of course. Still, it is important to note that depression or anxiety can have physical causes (a change in hormone levels or a side effect of some steroids), and these can and should be addressed by your doctor. Often a change in dosage of the medication can be helpful. In other cases, the depression or anxiety can be treated with specific prescriptions. Again, it is not a sign of weakness to address depression.

The fourth physical symptom, fatigue, can be a major issue for patients during chemotherapy or radiation therapy, recovering from surgery, or simply using energy to combat a cancer. Although many factors can cause the fatigue, dealing with the tiredness is possible. Most importantly, although you are aware that cancer treatment can make you tired, it is important to let your doctor know what you are experiencing. Make notes on how much sleep you get at night and during the day, how much fatigue impacts your daily activities, and especially if your fatigue suddenly or gradually worsens. Many underlying, treatable problems can be addressed if the health-care team knows about them. For example, a blood test can reveal anemia (low red blood cell count) which may need to be treated with iron supplements, stimulating factors, or transfusions. Radiation therapy in particular is known for causing fatigue. This is not your run-of-the-mill tiredness but a sometimes sudden loss of energy or physical stamina in the middle of routine activity. Listen to your body! Pace yourself so you have energy available for the most important parts of your day. Maybe you will choose a rest in the morning before the children come home from school. Maybe you will cook dinner in the morning when your energy is highest.

An important part of your physical well-being is your immune system. Boosting it is now recognized as an integral part of the treatment of cancer. The current belief is that each one of us, at any given time, is living with one or more rogue cancer cells or clumps of cells but that they usually don't become a problem because they are eradicated by our white blood cells. A subgroup of the white blood cell population, the T-cells or "killer" cells, recognize foreign cells that are not supposed to be in our body and attack them. This leads to cancer cell death and a return to normal body functioning. Sometimes the T-cells do not do their work, or they are overwhelmed by the size of the tumor. At this point a clinical cancer may be detected.

Given this picture, it is important to do everything you can to stimulate the activity of the T-cells and to keep your immune system active against bacteria and viruses as well. What are some of the things that can strengthen the immune system? You might be surprised! Adequate sleep, rest and exercise help. Diet plays an important role. Mental activities such as meditation and visualization have been shown to have a measurable effect on T-cell activity. Physical treatments including Reiki, yoga, tai chi, and acupuncture can also boost immunity. Avoiding stress or learning how to manage it effectively is crucially important.

How does illness affect our mind, our **mental** fitness? Any illness, even the flu, demands our attention and interferes with our ability to think things through. Grieving, which is a normal part of the diagnosis of a major illness, can cause confusion and the sense that "I just can't think." In addition, medications can alter our thought processes by making us sleepy, jumpy, or depressed. For someone with cancer, an additional challenge can be what is lightly referred to as "chemo brain." Not every cancer patient receives chemotherapy and not every chemotherapy agent has the same effect on the mind. It is useful to know that this is a possibility, however, so if it occurs you can ask your doctor about possible alternative medications. Most importantly, it is reassuring to know you are not unique, you are not going crazy, you are not "weak," you are simply experiencing a side effect of your treatment. For many years this side effect was not acknowledged and patients just stumbled along doing their best. Now chemo brain is a clearly recognized clinical entity. It most often manifests in a sense of being in a bit of a fog, overwhelmed, like a computer that simply cannot process all the data at once. Not only is there an exceptional amount of data to process, but the stakes are huge, leading to additional emotional pressure. Confusion can be intermittent. You may have problems prioritizing—it can seem that everything demands attention at once, now! Memory impairment can occur, especially in short-term memory. Your sense of time can be distorted so nights seem to drag on forever while happy times are fleeting. Problems with memory, concentration, and executive function can lead to worry. Inability to multi-task can require you to start over after an interruption or distraction. Learning takes more effort and more time.

Can anything be done? Some medications may be helpful. Exercising regularly is one of the best ways to clear the fog, and it will help with worry and stress, too. Get adequate rest. Coping strategies such as writing notes to yourself can take over some of the automatic remembering that used to happen effortlessly. Some of the tools intended to help those with memory problems can also help you— you can find these at a drug store. The pill sorters that group medications by date and time of day can provide a visual reminder of whether you did or did not take your medication this morning. Some devices have timers with alarms to remind you to take your next dose. You can post a calendar to write down appointments and important health habits including walks or stretches. In most cases this disturbance in thinking is temporary and will ease with time and the end of treatment, but some patients face continuing challenges.

Once you are confident that your physical self is getting the most ideal treatment possible, consider your **emotional** state. Even with adequate sleep, pain control, and treatment for anxiety, you may still find yourself an emotional wreck! This is usually the result of so many things requiring your attention simultaneously. You may be feeling depressed about the weather, sad about losing a job, grieving about the loss of your healthy future, scared about money, and lonely. We are so accustomed to having a sense of predictability about our future! From our earliest days, we have written a script in our minds for how our "ideal" life will proceed. Suddenly the script has been torn from our hands and we face a future filled with uncertainty. We no longer make plans for a trip in five years—we may not be here then! Even short-term planning can be disrupted by factors beyond our control: a fever, a cold, a broken bone, a "bad day."

It requires a major change of outlook to accept this new reality. In fact, it isn't a "new" reality, it's just that for the first time we recognize the unpredictability of our future. No one knows what lies ahead, what blessings or challenges may await us. Our opportunity now is to decide how to frame our thoughts, how to come to inner peace with the fact that we just don't know, and can't know, and never will know. As children we have a mythical belief that when we become "grown up" we will have answers for every situation. One of the blessings of aging is recognizing that no one has all the answers, and all of us are just muddling along the best we can.

This is not to say that nothing can be done! This battle in our mind and heart can be supported in many ways. Tools are available, but we may be unfamiliar with them because we have never used them before. We can be empowered by our illness to discover new and healthier ways of coping with life.

Coping with fear can be the most difficult part of the cancer journey. Fear is a part of almost every patient's experience. You are not alone—all of us, patients and caregivers alike, struggle with fear at one point or another. Fear does not go away by being ignored. We can minimize its impact on us by facing it! Unresolved fear uses up emotional, mental, and physical resources and robs us of hope, joy and strength for today.

"Fear work" is a long-term commitment, not a one-time effort. The first step is to identify what it is you fear. Maybe it is global, "I am afraid of the whole situation!" Maybe it is fear of death, or losing independence, of leaving work unfinished, of the sorrow your loved ones will feel as they see you decline. Finances are a big fear and often a big unknown. You may face fear of losing your job, your role in the family, your reputation, your self-image—the list is pretty much endless. We can be worriers! Likely you will check off several of these fears as ones you share. What next?

Set aside a time when you are rested and will not be interrupted to do some "fear work." (See Chapter 3.) Don't do this at night, when fears become larger than life! Grab some paper and a pencil and look at the things you fear. Write them down, write down what would happen if that fear became reality, and list your options if that happens. A fear named is a fear tamed!

Information can empower you to face fear. But beware! Too much information or the wrong kind of information (that which doesn't apply to your situation) can be harmful to your emotional health! It is always best to ask your doctor about the things you fear—some may not apply to you at all. You can also seek assistance from professional caregivers, medical personnel, faith-based counselors, or social workers. Good sources of information you can rely on are the American Cancer Society and the National Cancer Institute. Both have twenty-four-hour hotlines staffed by real people.

Something to consider: Courage is not the absence of fear but proceeding in spite of it!

Emotional instability can be a part of your journey. We often don't realize how much energy it takes to "filter" our emotional responses to the demands of daily life. We may be grouchy! You may have a decreased tolerance for noise, confusion, changes in routine, or physical clutter or disorder. Patients want to be on "autopilot," able to walk safely around their home without worry about tripping over clutter or an unfamiliar arrangement of furniture.

While we are busy working on our physical, mental, and emotional fitness, we are simultaneously faced with other people in our lives. You may discover that relationships and social engagements look very different while you are ill. The **social** aspect of our health isn't just incidental; it is an intrinsic part of who we are as members of families, churches, schools, and communities, and it needs to be addressed. Responses vary. Some people withdraw completely and cease to interact with the outside world at all, while others thrive on activity and the energy and support they receive from others. You are still the same person you were before your illness. If you have always been a loner, you probably won't change radically into someone who loves a crowd, but this is a good time to re-evaluate the place of other people in your life.

The most important person or people are those we call "care*givers*." This broad term covers everyone who cares for and about you—your doctors, nurses, therapists, family members, neighbors, and friends. It becomes evident rather quickly who makes you feel cared for. Seek out these people! Spend more time with them. Thank them and invite them along on the journey you are taking. Their support can give you added strength just by their encouragement. If they also do chores, mowing your lawn or washing your dishes, that is a great bonus.

Other people in your life might be called "care*takers*." These are the folks who deplete your emotional reserves, the ones who come to you to make *them* feel better. Sometimes family members can fall into this category. They can create additional work for you by expecting you to carry on with business as usual, not realizing that changing sheets or preparing meals may require more strength than you have available. Sometimes these people are struggling with their own emotions about your illness and can't contain their sorrow, worry, or despair. Anyone who depletes your hope or makes you feel worse is a *taker*, not a *giver*. Avoid them! Let the answering machine take their calls. Explain that you are not up to a visit right now.

As the person coping with illness, you have the right and the responsibility to choose how you spend your time and which people you want to have near you. If you are a people-pleaser it may be an entirely new concept for you to take the risk of hurting someone's feelings to protect your own. It can be done. Practice a few deflecting comments so you will have the words available when you need them.

"I am really tired right now. I'm sorry I can't visit."

"I'd like to talk with you, but this has been a demanding day. Can we plan another time to talk?"

"I am focusing all of my energy on my health at the moment, and I need to spend time resting."

"I prefer not to talk about my illness but would rather focus on other topics."

What about your immediate family, the people who live with you? This illness will certainly change the dynamics in the household. Sometimes the breadwinner becomes a patient, sometimes the homemaker can no longer "make" the home. Life will change for all of you, whether you want it to or not. It is most helpful to establish an honest dialogue right from the beginning. Allow one another the chance to express feelings, even the negative ones. Unless there is open communication, unnecessary resentments build; misunderstanding becomes the norm, hurt feelings and misconceptions rule the day.

One helpful way to do this is to set a day and time (without interruption) to talk about your illness and the changes it will mean for the family. Include everyone. Allow plenty of time. Reassure everyone that there are no dumb questions. Let people know that you love them deeply and that you want most of all for this time you have together to be richer and more mutually supportive. Express what you will need in terms of physical and emotional support. Maybe this means regular meal times. Maybe you will require more quiet for resting. Perhaps you will want to set aside time for yoga, prayer, or meditation. Maybe you will need rides to treatments or therapy appointments. If you spell out what you will need, you give your loved ones the opportunity to meet those needs and do their part to make the household run smoothly.

This communication is especially important to children, whether young or adult. It is a very scary experience for any child to witness a sick parent. The very young may think they caused the illness or be afraid of catching it. They may misunderstand a prognosis. Their fears are only magnified if the parents don't include them in the information sharing. If each person can rely on the others to be honest as the journey unfolds, each can be calm in the face of whatever storms might lie ahead. If problems are hidden to "protect" someone else, the protected person loses trust in the relationship and believes they are not important enough, or that you don't believe in them enough, to share the truth. Honesty may not always be easy, but it is right. (For more on the topic of family, see Chapter 4, Cancer as a Family Affair.)

Spiritual health is the last, but by no means the least, aspect of our overall wellness. Soul pain is as real, and maybe more distressing, than physical pain.

Spirituality means something different to each one of us. For some, spirituality is expressed through a mainstream religion: Christianity, Judaism, Buddhism, or one of the many other faith traditions. For others, spirituality is more a matter of world view, connecting to nature or the outdoors. Each of us, in whatever way we are called, is a spiritual person, even if our belief system says that "this world is all there is." That, too, is a belief.

In the general course of living, spiritual matters can be put on a "back burner" and not considered since everything is going fine at the moment. We think we are too busy, tired, scared, or inadequate to consider matters of belief in an afterlife or the place of faith in our lives. Cancer has a way of shaking us out of our complacency.

Faith can play an important part in wellness. It is comforting to know there is a God who cares for you, personally, and will help you through your challenges.

Many cancer patients experience a more profound sense of spirituality as they deal with their illness.

When talking about spiritual matters, patients often refer to the power of prayer. Some prefer to call these "affirmations." Whatever they are called, the essence of this interaction is to tap into the connection between patients and their "higher power." It is recognized as an important spiritual coping mechanism by my "panel of experts" and is a place to turn when you feel you are at the end of your rope. Another theme that comes up over and over again is that patients can feel and actually experience the power of being prayed for by others. They feel a tangible, real presence of comfort in the midst of trouble that defies other explanation. Faith practices such as formal prayer, church services, meditation, yoga, or contemplative prayer can bring calm and centering in the midst of the chaos of treatment. They can provide an anchor to the eternal in the midst of a tumultuous "now."

One patient told me that she uses sticky notes throughout the house to remind her of the importance of her thoughts. Her favorites are, "I am happy, healthy and whole," "I can do all things through Him who strengthens me," "Accept and forgive." Other patients enjoy a daily meditation from a book of reflections, attend Mass, or offer the day to God.

One particularly powerful exercise of spirituality is to offer your suffering for the intention of someone you love who is in need. This spiritual support is a blessing to them and a reminder to you that although you may be ill, you can still make a difference in the lives of those you love.

One patient said, "I say my mantra, which I repeat several times a day. 'Thank you, Lord. I am in perfect health.' I told myself that I was in perfect health even when I was hanging on by a thread trying to survive until treatment could start."

Another remarked, "I don't expect a miracle but I believe in them. I pray. I let go and let God."

Cancer patients recognize that they will soon be entering eternity. This is true for all of us! Some believe life ends, is over, at the point of death. There is a vast array of beliefs about the afterlife. Many believe this one life will continue either in heaven or hell. Others believe in reincarnation. Whatever your personal belief, this is the time you will find yourself asking questions and seeking answers. All of a sudden it seems so important to get your spiritual house in order. It is good to consult with members of your faith tradition or spiritual directors to help with this process if you would appreciate assistance. Many hospice programs offer chaplains or spiritual care as well.

In short:

- Physical challenges can be addressed if your doctor knows what is happening.

- Mental changes are an expected part of the treatment and coping tips can ease the way.

- Emotional challenges can be intense and require

attention and compassion for yourself and those you love.

- Challenges often lead to spiritual growth.

Adding Alternative or Complementary Care?

⚜

Many readers have already searched for their "ideal" treatment and have made their treatment decisions. If you are comfortable with your choices, please disregard the rest of this chapter. If you are still wondering or are plagued by doubts, read on. You may want to re-read Chapter 17.

A question that is common to everyone who is living with cancer as a chronic condition is, "What am I missing? Have I really tried everything that is available? What is the latest, greatest treatment?"

The good news (and the bad news, too) is that it is pretty much impossible to be certain you have tried everything. Life is filled with uncertainty and what is accepted today may be disproved tomorrow. Don't beat yourself up over this! All any of us can ever do is to explore reasonable options, ideally with caregiver input, and then choose what makes the most sense for us here and now. No treatment comes with guarantees for cure or even for improvement, but many are available that can give some relief and may improve outcomes. How do you search for these, and what are the pitfalls?

First, be vigilant. Be aware that you are more vulnerable than usual and that unscrupulous clinics or "cancer groups" may target you. There are long-standing differences of opinion between providers of mainstream care (surgery, chemo, and radiation) and those who offer alternative and complementary care. Each side thinks the other is only telling part of the story, and that is actually pretty much true. The **traditional oncology** approach is strictly evidence-based; that is, the treatments are the result of carefully organized clinical trials that compare patients who receive different treatments, chemo agents, or radiation doses, using large numbers of patients and double-blind studies. (Neither the doctor nor the patient knows which regimen they are getting.) Once the studies are completed, the data are collected and the two study groups are compared in terms of side effects, tumor shrinkage, and length of life. This system follows the scientific method and has been the standard of care for modern medicine.

The **alternative** approach assesses each patient individually and develops a treatment plan based on the needs of that particular person, the kind of cancer they have, and their overall health picture. (Alternative therapy is used *instead of* traditional therapy, which is why it is called alternative rather than complementary.) Some of the treatments that may be offered are nutritional regimens, acupuncture, massage, yoga, Reiki, high-dose vitamin supplements, cleansing procedures, and new methods of delivering chemotherapy to the tumor. Most often several treatments are given simultaneously, so it is difficult to compare responses between patients. The treatment result is often referred to as anecdotal. That doesn't mean it isn't true or real, just that it can't be summarized statistically. If improvement results, it is not possible to determine which factor(s) were the ones that made the difference. The same is true if the cancer worsens.

Experimental research is rarely attempted in the fields of alternative and complementary care. Each patient receives many different interventions and because practitioners believe that everything works together for the patient's benefit, treatments vary widely from patient to patient.

Traditional providers often dismiss alternative treatments as unproven and inferior to standard care. Alternative providers believe that chemotherapy and surgery assault the body by damaging the immune system and make it more difficult for alternative treatments to be effective.

What is a patient to do? How can you decide?

1. Listen to your gut. Ask yourself if you, as an individual with your unique background and cancer, are drawn to one route or another. Start there.

2. Gather information. Please consider the source. The Internet is an extremely powerful tool, but the information available is only as good as the source (see bibliography). Who is the author of the site? What are his or her credentials? Not everyone who calls himself a doctor is one! Most importantly, are they

selling a product or service or are they sponsored by a pharmaceutical company or a cancer organization? Do you need to pay to access information?

3. Get your questions together. Once you have an idea of what might be helpful to you, write down the specific treatments you believe might help you and ask your doctor for input. You might feel awkward doing this, but it can help you determine both the validity of the complementary treatment and the open-mindedness of your doctor. You may find that this step will remove many of the complementary treatments as options because they are not appropriate for you. You may also find that your doctor is supportive of complementary treatments that can make you feel better during standard treatment. You may decide that you need a second or third opinion.

4. Once you have narrowed your choices, call the American Cancer Society hotline or the National Institutes of Health hotline and speak to an expert who has access to the latest papers written and information available. See what that person has to say.

5. Decide for yourself, in consultation with your caregivers. This really is your decision, and you will be living with the consequences for better or worse. It's your body! Your goal is to find the path you believe is best for you as a whole person, not only for the treatment of your cancer. You need to consider cost,

stress, travel demands, and disruption of your daily life. But remember that any time delay before beginning traditional treatment may prevent these proven treatments from working most effectively.

In short:

- Traditional care has been proven through scientific methods of study.

- Adding complementary care to traditional care can make you much more comfortable and happier.

- Many unproven but helpful interventions can ease the challenges of your illness and treatments.

- **Beware!** Not every "natural" intervention is harmless!

- The American Cancer Society and the National Institutes of Health offer guidelines to help you decide on the best care possible (see bibliography for Internet resources).

Breaking News and Treatments in the Works

Treatment for chronic diseases is a growing and rapidly changing field. It would be impossible to list every new procedure or promising medication or chemotherapy—but that is good news! A great deal of time, energy, and money are being devoted to improving care. What are some of the things to watch for?

One of the most promising fields of research is fueled by the results of the Human Genome Project. For the first time ever, you can be tested with a blood or saliva sample to discover your entire genome—the sequences of genes in your DNA that are responsible for everything your body does. Many mutations (which a person is born with) are associated with increased chances of developing a particular disease, including cancer. The BRCA1 and BRCA2 genes are probably the best known of these markers. As research continues, more and more DNA sites will be linked to illnesses. This will allow individuals who carry those genes to receive more specific screening for problems before they are symptomatic. A positive marker means there is a *tendency* to develop cancer at a greater rate than in the unaffected population. It is not a certainty! It does require vigilance and appropriate action. Prophylactic treatment aimed at reducing risk for an individual must be carefully weighed. Some patients are good candidates for mastectomy, hysterectomy, or colectomy based on their genetic makeup. Others may decide to watch and wait. These are important, high-stakes, personal decisions that must be made on an individual basis.

Additional genetic news includes the testing of one specific tumor (yours!) to see the changes in tumor DNA. Many tumors have changes in the cell wall that make them more or less susceptible to chemotherapy agents. Some have a specific receptor on the cell wall that can allow treatment with an agent that will selectively target your tumor and have less impact on normal cells elsewhere in the body. Some process chemicals in a way that can enhance or erase the effect of a drug. All of this means that you have an increased chance of receiving a drug that is most effective for your tumor and can spare you from receiving a treatment that will be ineffective.

Targeted therapies use the specific antigens on the surface of your cancer cells as targets for antibodies that are specific for your tumor. This is a form of immunotherapy, which helps your immune system fight cancer. The immune system is our healthy body's defense against both cancer and infections, and boosting that system or enlisting its help can direct the treatment to target only the tumor cells while sparing normal tissues. The result is fewer unwanted side effects! Your own tumor cells are isolated. In the lab, antibodies are produced which bind to the antigens in your cancer cells. These "monoclonal antibodies" bind to the specific tumor cells when they are reintroduced into your body in the form of therapy. They work to "deliver" either a chemotherapy agent or a radioactive chemical that will kill the tumor cells. Because these are specific for the tumor, they do not attack normal surrounding cells. This treatment has been especially promising for melanoma.

Another promising line of research involves production of "treatment vaccines" to boost the immune system's response to cancer cells. (These are not to be confused with the vaccines used for prevention of bacterial diseases.) Blood is removed from the patient, treated to recognize tumor cells, and re-introduced with antibodies for the tumor.

You may hear the term "angiogenesis inhibitors." What are these? The formation of new blood vessels (angiogenesis) is controlled by chemicals which allow for the repair of damaged vessels and the formation of new ones. Tumors must constantly produce new blood vessels in order to acquire oxygen and nutrients. Angiogenesis inhibitors are agents which interfere with the production of new blood vessels. These agents inhibit the growth of blood vessels to the tumor rather than directly attacking tumor cells. They don't necessarily kill tumors but may prevent them from growing. The agents may need to be given over a long period. The side effects can include bleeding, clots, and hypertension, and the possibility of impaired wound healing, heart, and kidney function.

Certain cancers are influenced by the blood levels of hormones such as estrogen, progesterone, and testosterone. This is especially true for breast cancer, ovarian cancer, and prostate cancer. In these cases, part of therapy may include medications to either increase or decrease levels of the hormones. This is not chemotherapy but acts to address the overall levels of hormone in the body.

Cyber-knife radiation/surgery is an advanced technology to treat cancer with radiation. The newest machines allow precise positioning of the radiation beams so that they can be focused directly on a tumor with less scattering to normal surrounding tissue. The radiation is provided all at once, rather than over several treatments with lower doses of radiation.

Adjuvant therapy refers to a combination approach which may include several drugs, chemo treatments, surgery, radiation, and sometimes complementary care to achieve greater results than one treatment by itself.

It is good to remember that not all low-grade cancers require aggressive treatment. In some cases the treatment may be more dangerous than living with the disease. Often a "watch and wait" approach is in your best interest.

In short:

- New discoveries allow for treatment with immunotherapy, hormonal therapy, angiogenesis inhibitors, and targeted therapies, as well as conventional chemotherapy, surgery, and radiation.

- Many cancer treatments are given in combination for best results.

- Treatment decisions are based on the individual tumor type, which varies from person to person.

What is a Clinical Trial?

Most new chemotherapy agents or treatments must be approved by the FDA as safe and effective before they are offered to doctors for use in patient care. The only way this can happen in the case of cancer is for current patients to be willing to try something new. This is an act of love, for yourself and for the patients who follow you. It may mean that your life is extended, your tumor goes into remission, or your symptoms ease.

What do you need to know to decide if this is the right choice for you?

First, you will need to qualify for the study. Each study has specific requirements. Some are for those with just one kind of tumor, some for people who have failed other chemotherapies, some for those who have had, or not had, radiation. The study may specify age limits, health limits (diabetes, heart conditions), or restrictions on your distance from the main study site. These requirements are usually technical and will probably need to be evaluated by your doctors. Almost always you will be closely monitored to see how the treatment is working. This may involve additional blood tests, scans, or physical measurements, performed either at the research site or your local facility. It is a two-edged sword. You will have additional interactions with the health-care system, but you will also have greater scrutiny, which can benefit you.

The purpose of the research is to compare different kinds of treatments. A study may compare a new agent to a placebo (something that looks like a medication but is inert), two different agents, or several agents already known to be effective to see if they can work even better in combination. The "gold standard" for a clinical trial is a double-blind study. That means that neither the patient nor the doctor knows which treatment any given patient is receiving. Only at the end of the study do the researchers compare the effects and decide if the new treatment is superior to the old way of doing things.

As a patient, you will want to know what phase clinical trial is being offered. Phase 1 trials are to evaluate safety and determine side effects. Phase 2 trials evaluate dosages. Phase 3 trials are for drugs that have already proven to be effective. They compare the new drug to standard care. Once in a while a new drug will be so promising that the study is discontinued so that everyone can have access to this improved treatment! In general, Phase 1 trials are the most risky to you since less is known. Phase 3 trials most often include one "arm" with the current most-effective treatment and one with the new, promising treatment in addition to the standard one.

You will not know and cannot choose which treatment you will receive. You will be assigned a group at random.

If you are interested in a clinical trial, let your doctor know. He or she will probably be aware of trials that may be a match for you. All clinical trials must be registered with the National Cancer Institute (ClinicalTrials.gov). The information at this site is provided by the study sponsor or principal investigator and does *not* necessarily reflect endorsement by NIH. You can search their web site by the type of tumor to see if any trials look promising for you. Go to www.cancer.gov/clinical trials search form. If you see something in the news or when doing your research that sounds interesting, it is always appropriate to ask if you might be a candidate.

Be sure to find out if your additional medications, treatments or visits will be paid for by the sponsors of the trial—they usually are. This is important because your own insurance may not cover any treatment considered "experimental." Legitimate researchers rarely, if ever, charge patients to participate. If there are fees to you, that is a red flag about the validity of the trial.

In short:

- You may be a candidate for a clinical trial, but the requirements are usually very specific. Check with your doctor to see if you qualify.

- A clinical trial can be both a great benefit to you and a gift to future cancer patients.

- Do your homework to discover the trial's phase, costs, and possible benefits.

Updated Job Description

All of us, over the course of our lives, make up a "job description" for ourselves. We need a guide, a compass, to get through the challenges of daily life and assure ourselves we are on track. This job description becomes a part of us, a piece of our identity and our world view. It is unique to each person, although a lot of the components are shared, especially in the same culture or generation. Often we don't even realize that we are making our life choices according to this script.

What might a job description include? It's my job to be sure I never disappoint anyone. I am the peacemaker. It's my job to keep my house clean. I need to attend each meeting. I must work all day, every day, because I have so much to do. I need to take care of others. I always run the company. I'm in charge of the finances. I'm the scoutmaster. I'm the host or hostess. I'm the person in charge of maintenance—car, house, yard. I step up to help with every project in my family, neighborhood or church. I will always do my part.

When we are facing a major life change such as the awareness we will be living with a chronic disease, it is necessary to rewrite the job description. What? That is WHO I AM! A gut reaction refuses to admit this need for change.

It is a little death, this letting go of the way things used to be. It is scary—if I change the job description, who will I be then? What will I have left?

It's important to make a distinction between what you *do* and who you *are*. What you *do* is variable, depending on the circumstances. Life offers us different opportunities to act; each day brings its own to-do list. Who you *are* is unchanging. It is the core of your being, the essence of your values, your beliefs, your self. When we rewrite the job description, we are merely changing the to-do list and not letting go of the person we are deep inside. One of the blessings of a time of illness is that the external or action-oriented tasks of our lives can fall away, revealing the inner self that has been hidden under all the activity all along. When ill, we are gifted with time to see this part of ourselves and to appreciate who we really are. We may meet ourselves for the first time and so may those around us. This is gift and grace. It brings freedom.

It can also feel unfamiliar, this openness to who we are. Our busy lives effectively mask our true selves, and we rarely sit and consider our inner essence. One of the gifts of illness is time—time to relax, time to think.

What is my life task? What is it for which I was created? What am I called to do during my time on earth? We are blessed with the big picture when we allow ourselves to consider it. The answers vary, of course. Maybe you will feel that your most important legacy is to raise your children to be responsible, productive members of their families and their world. Maybe you have developed a new idea—a product or a life view that you are called to share. Maybe you are a painter or poet, and you enhance the lives of those around you with this gift. Are you called to write? To speak your truth to others? To be a listener? To be a "freelance lover" who reaches out to those in pain? Perhaps you feel a call to pray for those in need around you, to spread your love wordlessly. When we identify what is most meaningful to our lives in the big picture, we can set out on the path of living in congruence with it. We can gain the satisfaction that we are truly doing our best in this crazy world to make it a better place, for ourselves and those around us. We can find peace.

In short:

- Evaluation and acceptance of new limits requires sometimes painful soul-searching.

- Willingness to build a new "job description" can lead to a peaceful heart and a sense of meaning.

Putting Your Affairs in Order

Have you ever stopped to think how many important pieces of information are stored in your own mind and nowhere else? Have you ever wondered what your husband or wife would do if you were suddenly unavailable to answer questions? In many families one member keeps track of the household business and the others are grateful to just go along without knowing even the basics about the running of the household or the finances.

If you become unable to answer questions, what are the important details for your loved ones to know? Figuring this out can be a daunting task: If you are not up to doing it now, you can verbally instruct a helper or family member to do this organizing for you, or even use a tape recorder to leave the most important facts. (You may prefer to come back to this chapter at a later date, when you are fresh and ready to address it.)

Maybe the most immediately necessary information relates to your financial system. Do you have a list of the bills you pay monthly? What are the recurring expenses? Do you have a folder or shoebox with the tax receipts and documents? Where are the tax returns from prior years? What outstanding debts do you have and what are the payment arrangements?

Where do you keep bank statements, life insurance policies, homeowner's insurance, car pink slips, and unpaid bills? Is the family credit card in your name? If any of this information is stored on a computer or is part of an automatic billpay system, be sure you leave access information, such as the password for your computer, the account name, the user ID, and the password for the account. Remember that anything on a computer will be useless without this information!

What are the directions for the household? Where are the warranties? How do you get the fan or heater to work? Where are the instructions for the power mower? What kind of maintenance is required for the car, the heater, the sprinkler system? How do you operate the washer and dryer?

Remember the legal papers—the lease or deed for the home, the marriage certificate and children's birth certificates, your will or trust documents.

Don't forget all the people you count on for assistance. Do you have a list with phone numbers of your banker, accountant, lawyer, financial planner, dentist, computer repair person, and the guy that comes to wash the windows or fix the plumbing? Organizing all of this information which is now in your head into a form that is logical, easy to find and reasonably complete will take a great load off your shoulders. It is a huge gift to your caregiver to know where everything is. It is one nagging worry you don't need and you will be delighted when the organizing is completed. *Getting it Together* is an excellent source to get you started so you don't feel completely overwhelmed by the task (see bibliography).

What about your "stuff"—belongings that are meaningful to you but won't mean anything to anyone else unless they know the story? Family heirlooms or sentimental jewelry or books fall into this category. Some families choose to indicate whom they choose to receive precious possessions by taping a note on the bottom of each piece. An even better alternative is for you to give as a gift the items that you know would bring pleasure to someone you love. You have the joy of seeing your precious belonging going to a person who is precious to you. You can tell the story—this belonged to Great Grandma or was received as a wedding gift fifty years ago. Many of our precious possessions continue to bring us pleasure just because we see them in our daily life. You can choose to keep these to enjoy now.

One very important part of putting your affairs in order is deciding on and putting in writing your wishes for your care at the end of your life. Again, this discussion tends to be avoided because it is human nature to think there will be a better time "later." Family members, or you, may be uncomfortable or embarrassed about your feelings when you discuss death. It is the elephant on the table that no one mentions and everyone hopes will just go away. It takes real courage to decide that this conversation is a priority for all of you. Fortunately a wonderful document can help with your planning. *Five Wishes* is available from the Aging With Dignity Foundation. It is short, written in common English (and available in many other languages), easy to understand, and comprehensive. *Five Wishes*, once filled out and witnessed (no lawyer or notary is required), is a legally binding document that is accepted by hospitals, physicians, and lawyers in every state except three. It allows you to designate the person you trust to make health care decisions for you if you are unable to speak for yourself. (This person is known as your Power of Attorney for Health Care.) You can explain, in advance, what kind of care you do or do not want if you are incapacitated. Do you want CPR? Do you want to be connected to a respirator or a feeding tube? Do you want your pain to be managed for maximum relief, or is it more important to you to be a bit more alert? One of the legal directives that comes up at the end of life is called "Allow Natural Death" (AND). This saves the patient and the family from the trauma of CPR, respirators, tube feedings, and emergency hospital admissions (see bibliography, *Hard Choices for Loving People*).

These are just a few of the issues you can discuss with one another *before* the information is needed. The biggest advantage to this preplanning is that you can be sure your family and doctors know very clearly what *you* want. You can prevent the heartache that occurs when loved ones are locked in battle because of their opposing convictions about what you want. It happens too often that brothers and sisters are fighting about what Mom wants rather than expressing their care and love for her as she lies dying. You can avoid this by clearly communicating *your* wishes.

The final piece of the organizing is a letter of instruction. This is your chance to talk to the people you love to ease their way through the challenges that anyone faces after a death. It can be as lengthy or succinct as you want. It needs to include the location of your important papers such as birth certificates and marriage licenses, military discharge papers, deeds, and pink slips. Be sure to give the name of the bank and the box number if you have a safe deposit box, or the opening instructions for any safe you use at home. Where do you keep the key or combination? There is a waiting period for access to a safe deposit box after a death, so items of immediate need should not be stored there: not a will, not a *Five Wishes* document, and not this letter of instruction!

The letter of instruction should include names of people to call immediately, such as dear friends, family members at a distance, the funeral home you prefer to use, and the Social Security department, if applicable. You will want to include the name and phone number of your executor, if you have chosen one (a good idea).

It can include personal wishes that may not be in a will. Do you want all the china to go to Mary and the hunting equipment to John? Do you want a specific heir to be able to live in your house if it becomes available? If you have young children, who do you choose to care for them?

Choosing a funeral home and/or cemetery plot can be very challenging, but the thought of it is worse than doing it! These folks are truly compassionate and understanding, and they are professionals at helping others face the choices. Are you willing to accept some discomfort now to ease the burden on your family at the time of your death? It can be greatly consoling for them not to have to guess whether you prefer cremation, a plain pine box, or an elaborate weather-proof coffin. Most family members just want to do what *you* would want, but you must find the courage to make your wishes known. During the discussion at the funeral home, address the financial picture, too. You may save a lot of money by prepaying or signing a contract in advance.

In short:

- Not one of us knows when our time on earth will be over.

- It is important for everyone, sick or well, to put affairs in order as a gift to those loved ones who will have to figure it all out.

- Knowing that you have made preparations will give you peace of mind that you have done all you could do.

Passing On Your Values and Wisdom

⁂

Part of the task for each of us during our lives is to consider what we will leave behind us, how the world will be different and better for our time here. If you have not done so, consider what impact you can make on the world, your city, your family, or your church. Keep a diary or talk about your experiences to those who can benefit.

When we consider who we are in our inmost being, we discover that this part of us is rarely spoken of or shared, even with those we love the most. Over the course of our life, we have developed a sense of who we are, what is important to us, and what we see as the meaning of our life. This is constantly being fine-tuned as the need arises. Events that can have a big effect on our soul are major life changes—marriage, the loss of a child, a divorce, a move, a new job, or an illness. We remain essentially the person we were born to be, but we also carry with us the accumulated wisdom and experience of our lives.

Our life has great value to us, our loved ones, and our world. If you had the chance, what advice would you give to those who follow you? What would you want to transmit from your heart to theirs? You will be the only one who knows what form this passing on of wisdom will take. It might be writing love letters for the future. It might be in the form of a statement of the beliefs that you hold dear. You might compose a blessing prayer. You may prefer an oral history which captures your story on tape or video (see bibliography, *Ethical Wills*).

This is an opportunity, not a "should do." You may decide that saying a simple "I love you!" says it all. That's beautiful. If you do choose to leave a more concrete expression of your love, you can be sure it will be treasured for years to come.

One act of love you might consider is to leave notes to your children or grandchildren to be given to them on special occasions—their graduation from high school, their wedding, or the birth of their children. You can preselect these cards and say how proud you are and how much they are still loved. You can include any tips you want, like "Savor this moment!" These cards can be placed for safekeeping with your letter of instruction, sealed and addressed to the recipient with instructions on when each card is to be opened.

In short:

- One of the most precious gifts you can give your heirs is the gift of your insights and values.

- You can consciously choose to share your soul with those you love.

Palliative Care or Hospice Compared to "Going it Alone"

❦

If you prefer not to deal with this topic right now, that's OK! Skip this chapter and know it is here for reference at a later date. If this is a timely concern for you or a loved one, be assured that you can discover how to live fully even as you are approaching the dying process.

This is a hot topic, a red-flag discussion for so many of us. Our American culture prefers to act as if life, young and healthy life, lasts forever. The media, the sports teams, the CEOs of large businesses, even the soccer moms expect that their lives will always look the way they look today. A cancer diagnosis or some other life-threatening health problem is often the first wake-up call that each one of us, "even me!" is mortal.

In the good old days, as family members needed assistance with health problems or simply old age, it was the norm for family or extended family to step right in and provide a rocker for Grandma by the fireplace. Families, even young children, dealt with illness and death at home as an expected part of life. With the advent of modern medical care, we have convinced ourselves that whatever is wrong with us *can* be healed, that we are *entitled* to healing, and that outcomes should *always* be ideal. If we are sick, we want everything that is possible done, even if that means time in a hospital or skilled nursing facility. Along with excellent medical interventions has come the superstition that speaking about death will somehow make it happen. Even physicians are reluctant to tell a patient or family member that someone is dying, in spite of everyone's best efforts. The unspoken attitude is that death is a failure. If that is so, we are all losers because truly we will all die!

When death approaches, if you have the blessing of a farewell time you have basically three options. You can **go it alone**—simply keep on keeping on. You can try harder, hurt more, "suck it up," and act as if nothing has changed. You can shut out the world and pretend that everything is OK, as it always was.

If you have chronic difficulties such as pain control, eating, or mobility issues, you may qualify for **palliative care**. This care is not intended to be curative but offers the skills of a dedicated team experienced in treating challenging problems for the long term. Palliative care is a fairly new specialty and is not available in all locations, but it is good to ask if it is an option for you.

If your illness would normally be expected to lead to your death in six months, you are a candidate for **hospice care**. Hospice? The very word strikes fear into many hearts, and far too many people see it as admitting defeat, giving up, or a death sentence. The reality is a whole lot friendlier!

The philosophy of hospice is that every person has the right to face death with dignity. Hospice workers can help you stay in your own home and receive the medical care you need. You can continue to be surrounded by those you love. Based on your unique situation, hospice can provide visiting nurses, meals, bathing assistance, housekeeping services, or respite for your primary caregiver. The people who work in this field have exceptionally loving hearts. It is not surprising that so many obituaries request that contributions be made to a hospice.

First of all, entering hospice care does not mean you are committed to it forever. Illnesses are unpredictable! You may discover that the excellent care you receive in hospice will actually improve your overall fitness and nutrition enough that you "graduate" from hospice because your prognosis has improved. Great news! Enjoy your new lease on life! If you change your mind and want standard treatments you can withdraw from hospice. It is always *your* decision.

Hospice care provides physical attention to ongoing problems such as tubes, wounds, anxiety, sleeplessness, and pain. For you, these medical challenges can seem scary and overwhelming. For hospice care providers, it is all in a day's work. They have chosen to specialize in this field, usually because they have a hugely loving heart! They provide specific protocols for treating constipation, breathing difficulties, pain, and mobility issues. These folks are experts. They will know what is the state-of-the-art treatment for you and will teach you and your caregiver.

The emotional support and the easing of stress for both patient and caregiver are powerful incentives. Some people are experiencing a loved one's death for the first time. They are unsure, frightened, and can feel very alone. Hospice workers are on call twenty-four hours a day, seven days a week. You can call in the middle of the night and speak to a real live person, not a message machine. Hospice workers, especially the social workers and nurses, can provide guidelines for the caregiver and empower him or her with the information needed in advance of a crisis. In fact, the goal of hospice is to *prevent* crises before they happen by providing adequate and patient-specific interventions to keep the patient comfortable.

Another big advantage of hospice is the availability of equipment to use. A hospital bed is a huge comfort to someone who needs to change position often but who is losing the ability to move easily. Sometimes a trapeze or a grab bar can make the patient more able to move independently and can save the back of the caregiver! Shower chairs and bedside commodes can add safety for those losing mobility.

Who pays for all this outstanding care? Good question! For those on Medicare, hospice coverage is usually 100 percent. For younger folks or those on private insurance, the details may change but the overall cost is almost always less than without hospice.

Does entering hospice care mean you have to leave home and go to a special hospice unit or house? No. Most often the decision for hospice is made with the intention that the patient will receive care and pass away peacefully at home, rather than in a hospital or facility.

Most people, when asked, will say that they would prefer to die at home. Most caregivers want to honor those wishes. When things are fairly stable, it is a doable plan. As the illness progresses and the patient becomes weaker and less able to participate in self-care, the burden on the caregiver can grow to the point that they say, "I just can't do this any longer." The options then become moving the patient to a care facility, hiring someone else to ease the load, or entering hospice care.

What is the time line? Should you wait until you really need the help before you find out about hospice? Any hospice worker will tell you that the care they provide is most helpful when it is started early, while the patient and caregiver are still living "normal" lives. This allows relationships to form between the hospice workers and the family, and everyone comes to know and respect one another. The patient has the opportunity to express desires. This foundation of trust is appreciated when things become tougher. The team can provide instruction in advance of a difficulty and even leave medications that can be used as needed.

What is the downside to hospice? In exchange for providing all the support needed for the patient at home, the patient agrees that he or she will not seek lifesaving procedures in case their condition worsens. This means no more chemotherapy, radiation therapy, or surgery with the hope of a cure. Radiation and chemotherapy can still be used if the aim is to increase the comfort of the patient, but everyone is aware that this is not curative. Oxygen can be continued if it is needed for patient comfort. Sometimes regular preventative medications—insulin or high blood pressure medicine—may be discontinued. If the patient suffers a heart attack or a stroke at home, the hospice team is called, not the ambulance.

Often as time grows more precious and energy resources become more limited, the patient or caregiver will decide to limit social contact to those most near and dear. The circle of people who intimately accompany the dying person can shrink. If you are a friend or even a family member, respect the need of the dying person to spend his or her spiritual and emotional energy where it is most valuable, on the transition ahead. Honor privacy and don't barge in, no matter how close you feel to the patient.

Excellent books (see bibliography) can explain what to expect as death approaches. When the patient and caregiver are prepared for the stages ahead, they experience less fear and more peace.

In short:

- Palliative care is available for those facing long-term disabilities or needs for pain intervention. It is not time-limited. Curative treatments can proceed simultaneously.

- Hospice care is available to patients with an estimated lifespan of six months. It provides a full range of physical, emotional, mental and spiritual support for both patient and family. Treatments with the intent to "cure" are generally excluded. The goal is patient comfort and quality of life for both patient and caregivers.

• Going it alone requires abilities and knowledge caregivers and patients usually do not have.

Asking For and Accepting Help

"What? I am the *helper*, not the one who has needs. How can I do this? I am strong and a giver, not a receiver." Oops! Your health has changed, and the size of your physical and emotional "bank account" has changed with it. You used to have ten hours of productive time a day, and now you might have two fifteen-minute windows for work. You used to be able to take on the burdens of the world, but now you are dealing with your own burdens that leave little left-over energy to help others. The Bible says it so well, "To everything there is a season."

This is your season to reap, to cast away burdens. Often in your life you have given without repayment, and gladly. This is the time in your life to allow others to give to you. Your time to pitch in to assist with needs around you may have drawn to a close, either temporarily or as a life change. You are, whether you like it or not, on the receiving end now. You can fuss, fume, and refuse to admit it, or you can gracefully accept it.

This does not mean you are weak! If you thankfully accept the gifts others want so much to give you, that itself is a blessing to them and to you. It is the way they, and you, can express your love for one another. This is the time to remember how much joy you felt when you were able to assist someone else who needed help. Didn't it lift you up to help a coworker before a deadline, to provide a meal, to visit someone who was hurting? Unless we recognize the value of helping for the *giver*, not only the *receiver*, we miss out on some of the greatest blessings of our lives. Bask in the joy of receiving! You may never have done so before, but this is an opportunity for personal growth in humility and gratitude, and for developing friendships, old and new.

As our society includes more and more people who are living with a chronic illness after medical interventions have saved their lives, we realize again the need to change our way of thinking. As a society, we are recognizing the value of the years after our intense, hardworking lives have eased. Millions of people live as survivors of cancer in the United States alone. Many others live with diabetes, congestive heart failure, epilepsy, or kidney disease. As our population ages and our medical care advances, more and more of us will be on the receiving end of care, at least some of the time. There are still, of course, many ways we can continue to *give* care—it may just look different now. As a result of this demographic shift, there is a growing recognition of the value of planning as part of receiving help.

It used to be that a mom with a new baby was showered with meals as she adjusted to her new life. The neighbors would gather to bring food to a family that had experienced a death. This short-term help makes a big difference. When folks are looking at long-term disability, though, having a system can be remarkably helpful. Some models are discussed in excellent books (see bibliography) and some are tailor-made by each individual. All begin with clear communication and a heart that is willing to receive.

You have probably already experienced people who want to help coming up to you or writing in a note, "Is there anything I can do to help?" Let's be clear. It is humbling to realize that often chores need doing, and you cannot do them all right now. The helping partnership begins with a clear statement of your needs. You may be embarrassed that you can no longer do these things for yourself. Don't be! You are not asking for help; it is being *offered* by someone who really wants to share your journey. You can do them and yourself a great service by accepting their offer.

One way to begin is to create a paper record for each individual or organization. List the things you need help with: rides to medical appointments, cooking/meals, shopping, prescription pickup, carpool assistance, yard work, house cleaning, and even companionship! Maybe you need more skilled help, such as assistance with dealing with medical bills or tax preparation, painting or carpentry work. Maybe you want to have someone go with you to medical appointments to provide a second set of ears and to record the advice of the doctor. Could a friend take over the meal-planning schedule so that you could count on meals three days a week, or on the day of a treatment when you are pretty sure you won't be up to cooking?

This written helper record should include name, address, best phone number, best time to call, and availability. List the things you need clearly and specifically: Prune the roses, water the garden daily, clean the toilets weekly, feed the animals when you are away. Clarify if advance notice is required or if you can just call any time, even at night. You can easily leave space for a checkmark for the tasks that appeal to your helper. If you ask each person who offers help to fill out this record, you will have a safety net for the unexpected. Keep these records in a place accessible to you and your home caregiver. When a need arises, for instance, when your driver to chemo comes down with the flu, you will have the ability to call and ask for help. Both of you know in advance that sometimes the helper will be unavailable and you have already given them permission to say no. Since they know they will have another opportunity to help down the road, they can refuse without guilt.

The system helps everyone. You know you have a backup for emergencies. Your helpers know they can plan to bring you dinner on Friday without worrying if you already have two other meals brought over that day. Your caregiver feels an easing of the concern of always having to be there for you. He or she is then able to pay attention to self-care needs. You are allowing members of your community to share the load of your illness, and you will be surprised how eager they are to do so. You will also be encouraged by how much stress is removed from your shoulders as you see the demands of daily living managed.

Don't worry about "How will I ever repay/thank you?" These people are happy to help, and their gift of service is given with no strings attached. A simple "thank you" from your heart will let them know you are grateful. Remember the days when you were happy to do the same kind of service for others? Now it is your turn to be a gracious receiver. Don't let the fear of writing unnecessary thank-you notes keep you from choosing to accept help!

In short:

- It is much more difficult to be a good receiver of help than a provider of help, but it makes a huge difference to both giver and receiver to be open to accepting help.

- A system can ease the challenge of organizing help offers.

- The humbling experience of needing help can make you a stronger, more compassionate person.

Caregiver Love

❧❦

Your caregivers—what would you do without them? These people have chosen to express their great love for you by assisting you with everything you need as your health declines. Your heart is full of gratitude—most of the time. Sometimes your heart is full of frustration! It is not easy caring for someone else, but you can help them by recognizing the challenges they face.

What are these challenges? Fear is a big one! They, like you, don't know the future and they may be struggling with the "what if's," especially the biggest ones: What if I can't do what is needed? What if I break down, physically or emotionally? What if I get sick, too? They clearly love you, or they wouldn't be caring for you, but they, like you, wonder if their care is enough to meet your needs.

Caring for your caregivers is a choice you can always make, regardless of the state of your health. Caring doesn't require doing, it requires listening and empathy. It is an attitude of the heart. You can give support to your caregivers in many ways.

Most important of all, insist that your caregivers take care of themselves! They have a most demanding job, one that they didn't choose—just as you didn't choose to be sick.

They are trying to balance meeting your needs with meeting their daily life demands (job, household, family) just as they did before this caregiving time. If they do not take care of themselves, they will become ill or depressed and then neither of you will benefit from the "generous" giving that exceeds what they can afford to give, physically or emotionally.

Plan for caregiver respite! Be willing to have someone else, maybe a friend or neighbor, or a hospice volunteer if you are at that stage in your illness, step in to care for you so your caregivers can do what they need to do. This can include exercise, napping, and personal care such as doctor appointments, haircuts, and dentist appointments. It is also important that your caregivers have someone to give them emotional support and a listening ear. This might be a counselor or social worker, a pastor, a support group, or a good friend. Caregivers need a chance to express fear and frustration to someone besides you! They don't want to burden you with their concerns, but those concerns are real and need attention. Encourage time away from you for a lunch with friends or a change of scenery.

Remember to express your thanks. This can be a spoken "thank you" or a nonverbal—but much appreciated—hug or squeeze of the hand. Be kind; ask gently, not crossly, for their help. Try not to take your frustrations out on them, even though they may be the only ones nearby.

Remember that their life has greatly changed, too. Put yourself in their shoes and see the tasks added to their daily life. Recognize the time and emotional demands they are trying to juggle. Realize that most of us, most of the time, are doing the best we can. Don't expect perfection! It isn't their job, and it is impossible, to meet your every need. They are only human, and sometimes they get overwhelmed, just as you do.

How can caregivers deal with their own inevitable frustration? From the point of view of the caregivers the demands can seem enormous. It seems they just sit down when you need something more. They may offer a meal and be refused, then asked for food half an hour later.

A note to caregivers. It is important to realize that the patient's reality has changed. Habits we take for granted, such as sleep or eating routines, become jumbled. His or her physical and emotional state can change quickly—fine one minute, exhausted the next. The plans you made yesterday may be cancelled at the last moment. Make plans anyway! If you can step into the shoes of the patient, you will be more able to accept their ups and downs. Encourage the patient to tell you how he or she is doing, and understand that that can change from moment to moment.

Find an activity that allows you release from being constantly "on call." Watch a movie! Take up painting, or writing, or journaling. Read a great book. Nurture friendships with people who lift you up, who accept you, warts and all, who are not judgmental. Don't isolate yourself from the outside world. Your service comes into clearer perspective when you can see that caregiving is just part of your life, not all of it.

In short:

- Caregivers are a beloved and precious part of the cancer journey.

- The caregivers in your life deserve and appreciate your patience and expressions of thanks.

- It is the responsibility of caregivers to care for themselves, too, and it is your job to encourage them to do so.

In Summary

If all of this seems just too much, be reassured. It is overwhelming, but you have dealt with overwhelming situations before. Remember how you felt the first day of high school? Or the first night at home with a new infant? Or after the move to a new home, far away from familiar family and friends? It seemed there was SO much to learn, and there was. You discovered that you could rise to the challenge and grow through it. You are facing what is perhaps the greatest challenge of your life, and as history demonstrates, you will discover the strength and courage you need along the way, step by step. No one figures it all out once and for all. Your needs are constantly changing and evolving and you will adapt and learn. You will be amazed at the abundance of love and caring in the world. You will give precious lessons to those you love.

Words are powerful. So often people hope for a cure, and that is wonderful, but not always attainable. Healing, however, is available to all of us. That is the result of doing the best we can as we grapple with our illness. Healing involves coming to peace with both our abilities and our limits, in spite of our cancer, and discovering the way to live fully the time we have been given.

I have saved the best for last. The following endpiece I discovered during my chemo days when I was feeling vulnerable and inadequate. It brought me peace and steadily increasing hope for a better me tomorrow. May it bless you.

Daily Survival Kit for Serious Illness

by Thomas L. McDermitt
A long-time cancer patient and skeptic

(You don't have to agree with all of this all of the time. But if it generally speaks to you, try to read all or parts of it every day, or have it read to you. Part of the help is in the doing, regardless of your attitude or emotions on that day. On some levels the help is gradual and often not evident.)

Today I am going to try to live through this day only, and not dwell on or attempt to solve all my problems at once; just focus on the piece that is today. I can do something for several hours that would be difficult to even think about continuing for several months.

Just for today, I am willing to accept the possibility that there is a purpose to this suffering; that it can be a source of meaning and growth for myself and others, though I may not always recognize the ways. And it seems possible that this suffering will not be in vain, because of what may be some kind of existence beyond.

Just for today, let me remind myself that I am basically a worthwhile person, worth loving, despite my faults and limits. I deserve the efforts of others to help me through my illness.

Just for today, I want to be aware that it is all right to want too much from others at times. Illness brings out and intensifies the small child in all of us. And if I feel hurt when those who care for me cannot be there, it may help to remember that they have needs, frailties, and limitations of their own. A lack of response does not mean that they are personally rejecting me.

Today I may feel the need to complain a great deal; I may have little tolerance; I may cry; I may scream. That does not mean that I am less courageous or strong. All are ways of expressing anger over this mess, of rightly mourning my losses. Endurance itself is courage.

It is my life at stake now. So maybe today I can allow myself to be a little less concerned about the reactions or impressions of others. Maybe I can allow myself to feel a little less guilty or bad about what I did not accomplish or give. Perhaps today I can be a little more gentle toward myself.

Surviving this is all so difficult. At times it seems impossible—that I have had enough. Down the line I will know if and when I have had enough, when I cannot push the limits any further. I will have the right to choose to stop, without feeling that I am "giving up." But today I think I can deal with this illness. Sorrow runs very deep, but I think I can rise again.

Just for today, maybe I can give healing "the benefit of the doubt." The drugs are powerful; the natural healing capacity of my body is powerful. And who knows, perhaps there is healing power in my will to struggle, and in the collective love and will of others.

Just for today, perhaps I can take heart that we are all connected. And I may still have some things left to contribute to the family of man; some light to add to the light. Even now my endurance (however imperfect) is a gift, an inspiration for others in their struggles.

It seems reasonable that there is a season for everything, and a time for every purpose. Pain, weakness and exhaustion may distort my senses and spirit. Today, however, I can at least find some hope in nature's way, if not in some master plan. The chances are fairly good, and it seems worthwhile to hope that I will have some cycle of wellness yet.

©1989 by Thomas L. McDermitt
(Used by permission of GlaxoSmithKline, who bought the copyright.)

Bibliography

General Guides

Five Wishes: The DVD: America's Favorite Way of Planning for and Discussing Care at the End of Life, Available through Aging With Dignity.com

Caring for the Cancer Patient at Home, American Cancer Society

Ethical Wills: Putting Your Values on Paper, Barry K. Baines, M.D.

Share the Care, Cappy Capossela

From This Moment On, Arlene Cotter

Get It Together—Organize Your Records So Your Family Won't Have To, Melanie Cullen

The Seven Levels of Healing (available as DVD or book) Jeremy Geffen

The Measure of Our Days: A Spiritual Exploration of Illness Gerome Groopman, M.D.

The Anatomy of Hope: How People Prevail in the Face of Illness Gerome Groopman, M.D.

The Road Less Traveled, M. Scott Peck

Love, Medicine, and Miracles, Bernie Siegel

Radical Remission, Kelly A. Turner

Approaching death

The Four Things That Matter Most, Ira Byock

The Best Care Possible: A Physician's Quest to Transform Care Through the End of Life, Ira Byock

Dying Well: Peace and Possibilities at the End of Life, Ira Byock

Final Gifts, Maggie Callanan and Patricia Kelley

Hard Choices for Loving People: CPR, Artificial Feeding, Comfort Care, and the Patient with a Life-Threatening Illness, Hank Dunn

On Death and Dying, Elisabeth Kubler-Ross, M.D.

Living with Death and Dying, Elisabeth Kubler-Ross, M.D.

Facing Death and Finding Hope: A Guide to the Emotional and Spiritual Care of the Dying, Christine Longaker

To Die Well: A Holistic Approach for the Dying and Their Caregivers, Richard Reoch

Internet sites you can trust

Medlineplus: http://medlineplus.gov

National Institutes of Health: http://nih.gov

National Cancer Institute: http://www.cancer.gov

American Cancer Society: http://www.cancer.org

Fertile Hope: https://www.livestrong.org/we-can-help/livestrong-fertility

About the Author

Teresa Kalvelage Matthews is a twenty-three-year survivor of ovarian cancer and a twenty-year survivor of breast cancer. These two unrelated cancer "adventures" gave her a passionate dedication to easing the journey for other people facing similar challenges. A writer with a degree in biology from UC Berkeley, she has worked in medical office settings, as a hospice volunteer, and as a spiritual support volunteer. Her inspirational, hopeful, and practical tips provide a blueprint for people beginning treatment. Her insights into the patient's point of view have been used for professional training for hospice volunteers and social workers. She currently counsels newly diagnosed cancer patients.